DIET REVOLUTION

Nutrition, Diets, and Food Fads:
What the Experts Haven't Told You

DIET REVOLUTION

Nutrition, Diets, and Food Fads:
What the Experts Haven't Told You

by

JILL WORDSWORTH

St. Martin's Press
New York

Copyright © 1977 by Jill Wordsworth
All rights reserved. For information, write:
St. Martin's Press, Inc., 175 Fifth Ave., New York, N.Y. 10010.
Manufactured in the United States of America
Library of Congress Catalog Card Number: 76-13046
ISBN: 0-312-21000-0

Library of Congress Cataloging in Publication Data

Wordsworth, Jill.
Diet revolution.

1. Nutrition.   2. Food additives.   I. Title.
QP141.W65   613.2   76-13046

CONTENTS

page

Introduction 9

CHAPTER

I The general idea *11*
II What makes us tick? *22*
III Who are the experts? *35*
IV Back to basics *51*
V Diseases of civilisation *64*
VI More about deficiencies *86*
VII More about poisons *120*
VIII What health foods have to offer *138*
IX Summing up *158*
 Bibliography *177*
 Index *181*

TO
K and C

ACKNOWLEDGEMENTS

THIS BOOK COULD not have been written without the help of the many patient people who gave time to answering my questions. I would particularly like to thank Miss Dorothy Hollingsworth of the British Nutrition Foundation and Mr Douglas Drysdale of the British Naturopathic and Osteopathic Association, who each put up with me for a whole afternoon, and Dr Walter Yellowlees, who gave valuable advice on Chapter II. Many others who helped with information in their widely differing fields include:

Mr Max Altman, Mr Richard St Barbe Baker, Lady Eve Balfour, Alan and Clare Claydon, Dr Michael Crawford, Dr David Davies, Dr T. P. Eddy, Dr N. Fisher, Mrs Dorothy Forster, Professor L. Galzigna, Dr Douglas Gibson, Mrs G. Gillett, Mr Maurice Hanssen, Mrs Kathleen Jannoway, Dr Barbara Latto, Mr Frank Lewington, Mrs S. Pettett, Mrs Miriam Polunin, Dr Magnus Pyke, Mr Ken Rusby, Dr Gerald Shaper, Professor Curtis Shears, Dr Hugh Sinclair, Mr Leonard Stocks, Mr Michael van Straten, and the staff of Enton Hall, Godalming, Champneys, Tring, the London Nature Cure Clinic and the British College of Naturopathy and Osteopathy.

J. W.

DIET REVOLUTION

Nutrition, Diets, and Food Fads:
What the Experts Haven't Told You

INTRODUCTION

A S P E C I A L I S T   W R I T E S : "One of the alarming aspects of the growing Health Food cult is the way people with no qualifications or experience have started to tell us what to eat, drink etc. . . ." Another more picturesquely puts it: "No one would trust himself to ride in a train across a bridge when both train and bridge have been built by self-styled experts with no engineering experience. But thousands of people are prepared to trust their bodies, their health and ultimately their lives, to any person who sufficiently loudly proclaims he is a nutritional expert."

Why, then, are thousands prepared to take this risk? Probably because the "self-styled experts" are pretty persuasive on paper, with plenty of logic behind their arguments (though some of it may be unscientific and over-simplified), and possibly because one of the strongest human instincts is hope. If life seems drab and your back aches, the dazzling vista of a fresh start via diet (or yoga, or meditation) comes like a promise of spring. By contrast the dull reiteration "You've never been better fed" has all the impact of a damp firecracker. When hope is the driving force, the establishment can't win.

But not all food reformers are unqualified engineers driving broken-down trains. Many are experts in their field. How do we pick the right ones? How do we decide when hope is justified, or when the status quo might be better after all?

Read half a dozen diet books and you may find a common thread woven through all of them, leading you to some cheerfull conclusion like "honey is good" or "sugar is bad". But more often you find a mass of contradictions, or more perplexing still, similar views arrived at for totally different reasons.

Then, to add fuel to the flames of confusion, there are one or two books by doctors, knocking the health food cult as hard as they can, lashing out at fringe medicine and quackery and possibly steam-rollering some perfectly reasonable theory in the process.

So what is the earnest reader to do? Usually one of two things. The more gullible latch on to the first diet theory they read about and become disciples, while the sceptical, the lazy and the confused give it all up in disgust and carry on eating as they always did. Perhaps a small minority may battle on, trying to sort out the wheat from the chaff, and it is for those few that this book is written.

I am not qualified to give a verdict, only to summarise the many rival theories which compete for our attention and to present them side by side, so that the reader can see who thinks what. As far as I know, this has not been done before.

Each chapter is followed by questions and answers. The questions are those which occurred to me when I first began delving into food reform theories, and which I imagine will occur to most people. The answers are a composite of food reform opinions in general; where they are minority opinions, I name the one who holds them. Perhaps if we ask questions from all angles and try to sift the evidence, a pattern may emerge. Maybe a diet dialogue can guide us through the maze of facts, fancies and fads that make up the food reform movement. Let's try it.

CHAPTER I

THE GENERAL IDEA

F OR Y E A R S W E ate what we liked or what we could get. Later, the idea of a balanced diet came to be appreciated, then early in this century vitamins burst on the scene. Since then we have become more and more diet conscious.

In the early years, those who found fault with the average diet—a very small minority—were regarded as cranks. First in the field were the naturopaths in Europe—mainly in Switzerland and Germany—whose ideas were studied and sifted by Gayelord Hauser during the 1920s and popularised throughout Britain and America between the wars, mainly by lectures.

Since World War II we have had a "diet explosion", with popular books pouring off the press in ever increasing numbers as the public realises that feeling like death most of the time and expiring in one's sixties can hardly be what our creator intended. Perhaps the shattering statistics of World War II draftees in the US forces (50 per cent unfit) had something to do with it.

Human nature likes to have a scape-goat. If we feel irritable, depressed, lethargic and are creaking in the joints we like to be able to blame it on something other than our treadmill existence with its monotony, stress and lack of exercise; so we blame our diet. The two big scape-goats this century have been (1) poisons, and (2) deficiencies.

Poisons came first. Way back in my childhood I remember the poison advertisements—a young lady holding a glass of fizz and saying "Inner cleanliness comes first", or a delightful old gentleman with a twinkle in his eye vaulting over a five

11

bar gate. Both these people got rid of their poisons by taking health salts, liver salts, fruit salts or whatever you chose to call the alkaline mineral drink which washed away those nasty acid residues that made you feel so terrible. It sounded a perfectly reasonable theory and the health sales business has flourished on it ever since.

Deficiencies came later, with increased knowledge of vitamins and the feeling on the part of many nutritionists that food processing was getting somewhat out of hand. Once again, human nature seized the chance of a short cut. Put back the missing nutrients, preferably in the form of a single pill, and the old folk will be jumping over gates again.

Where crusaders go, big business is not far behind. You name it, somebody will sell you something to fix your deficiency. A popular health magazine of 194 pages carries more than 120 advertisements, mostly for supplements. First came the single vitamins, then the multi-vitamins, then the minerals, now the whole lot together. In the background, repeating their creed monotonously, though not loudly enough to get much attention, are the doctors. Their story is: you get enough vitamins and minerals with your knife and fork in ordinary food; you don't need supplements under normal conditons. Doctors do prescribe vitamins and/or minerals for certain ailments, but it's their everyday use which they say is unnecessary. And, as with patent medicines, they say we're being taken for a ride. Those fancy extras cost about ten times as much as they should. As one wag has it, "the only mineral the worriers are likely to find themselves short of is silver."

Food reformers are not particularly in favour of artificial supplements either. But whereas most GPs deny that deficiencies exist at all, food reformers say they do, very much so, but the cure lies not in pills but in fresh, unprocessed foods, if you can get them. Only in the last resort should you take supplements.

Who are we to believe? Most of us, when sick, go to a doctor and trust blindly in his judgement. But at other times it is novelty which appeals—the new idea, the new discovery, the wonder food, the wonder pill.

Officially we are told we have never been better fed. (Cynics add . . . or worse nourished.) This claim is based on three things:

1. The tremendous variety of food now available which a generation ago was unknown. (Until I ate my first avocado in Africa in 1950, I had never seen one. Now, anybody who has not seen an avocado is a freak.) We are able to have a truly mixed diet and this in itself adds to the nutritive value.

2. The hygienic nature of food, brought about by improved technology and enforcement of regulations. It is rare to find anything in a shop that has gone bad; food poisoning cases are the exception; packaging ensures a minimum of handling; flies in a supermarket?—there's no future for them there.

3. The existence of a benevolent watchdog in the shape of the Food and Drug Administration which sees fair play. Have the vitamins been knocked out of something? Put them back in. Do the old folk get the right nutrients? Do school children need extra milk? Are additives safe? A sore point this, but despite the allegations of food reformers, there is official concern on the subject.

We take all this so much for granted that it is hard to visualise life without preservatives, refrigerators and plastic. But in past centuries food (unrefined and free from additives though it might be) was a potential killer. Rural people could harvest and eat or slaughter and eat without delay; town dwellers had to take a chance. "Morbidity and mortality due to food deterioration must have been a major factor during the Middle Ages," writes a scientist. Cover-ups were needed in the form of strongly flavoured sauces; spices (with a preservative value of their own) helped to disguise dubious dishes. Later toxic chemicals were added to deceive the consumer. It was not until microbiology became a science that the bugs behind food poisoning were identified and suitable preservatives were found. We have had "safe" food for a mere hundred years. All this gives scientists a justifiable sense of achievement so that the reformers' cry of "back to the good old days" is nothing but an irritation.

Food reform needs more than the emotional appeal of the past to gain support. It needs a realisation that the past was not all good, plus hard facts supported by scientific findings, and a means of getting these across to the public in the form of easy-to-read books. There is no shortage of easy-to-read material, but assessing its value is no simple matter.

Go into any health food store and you will usually find, in addition to foods and supplements, a bookshelf displaying paperbacks and magazines on all aspects of food reform. The main magazines also run their own publishing companies which publish, in addition to the magazines, books by their regular contributors. Amongst the remaining miscellany, there seems to be a correlation: the thinner the book, the greater the rubbish, for interspersed with much useful writing you find a few booklets one can only term junk, written by people with obvious lack of scientific knowledge whose ravings fully justify the epithet "muck and mystery" which has been hurled at the food reform movement as a whole.

If you buy one or two books you get a lop-sided viewpoint, since most of them are written by people on hobby horses. If you buy the lot you run out of time and money. So it is simplest to group the books, magazines and authors according to what they stand for, then the large number of titles begins to fall into a pattern.

The popular magazine *Prevention* was founded before World War II by the amateur American nutritionist and organic farmer J. I. Rodale, who despite having a hole in the heart, lived for over seventy years. The British version of the magazine is edited by his son, Robert Rodale. Rodale Press also publishes a monthly magazine *Organic Gardening and Farming* with a guide on the same subject *The Organic Food Finder and Directory,* and a vast number of books which are really collections of reprints from *Prevention*.

Perhaps the most persuasive individual writer on nutrition was the American, Adelle Davis, a professional qualified trailblazer with the gift of putting across a complicated subject entertainingly. She is pretty caustic on the subject of amateurs: "Food faddists and crackpots have kicked nutrition pretty cruelly. They usually have no scientific training, peddle tremendous amounts of misinformation, make unjustifiable claims and are often out for commercial gain. They not only put people off by their ridiculous recommendations, they make every thinking person necessarily sceptical of the whole subject."

Despite these strictures, Adelle Davis has herself been called a faddist by the medical profession who distrust her conclusions, and accused of the very practices she denounces, almost word for word. One critic writes: "Miss Davis has found it financially profitable to make a good story for food faddist preparations to the extent that she pays little attention to the accuracy of her subject matter." Davis yells back, "Who is paying for the research of the people who criticise me?" When you have heard some of the scurrilous things that scientists of opposing views say about each other, you realise that those exchanges are comparatively mild.

Amidst all this literature, two schools of thought emerge— the British (represented by Nature Cure) which tends towards vegetarianism, and the American represented by Gayelord Hauser, his slightly younger rival Lelord Kordel, and Adelle Davis, among others) which puts great emphasis on a high protein diet. Both, however, insist on whole foods and unite in condemning the refining business. More about these schools of thought in Chapter III. The layman can hardly be blamed for feeling baffled by the diverse subject matter thrust under his nose. But when you boil it all down to essentials, what we find are our two old friends, poisons and deficiencies, very often combined in one package.

The poison idea has changed quite a lot since the early days.

Then it was simply a matter of "auto-intoxication"—stay constipated long enough and you start re-absorbing the residue you ought to have got rid of—an idea never fully supported by doctors. Today, poisons are said to be rushing at us from many directions, some from the farm, some from the factory and some from inside our own bodies. But what exactly do we mean by poison?

Many of us think of poison as something that either kills you off or makes you so ill that drastic action by the doctor is needed. This kind of poison if eaten is rejected by the body long before it can be digested, so if you live to tell the tale you have got rid of it. It is the build-up of tiny quantities of wrong things day after day for years which food reformers are worried about, because the results may not be recognised as directly connected with eating habits. The poison hazards are said to be these:

1. Poisons from insecticides, weed killers and so on which get into plant foods, plus poisons from the growth-promoting hormones and anti-biotics given to domestic animals which may be toxic in themselves or may lead to chemical reactions we know nothing about. Food reformers say the answer is to revert to naturally produced food. (See Chapter IV.)
2. Poisons from additives which have not been adequately tested. These include artificial colourings, flavourings, improvers, preservatives and so on. The answer, according to food reformers, is to eat foods which have not been tampered with, which health food stores claim to sell.
3. Poisons which are the result of a faulty diet—either eating too much, eating refined foods, or eating normal foods in the wrong proportions. This is the special hobby horse of the Nature Cure people, who also regard medicines as poisonous. More about their theory in Chapter III.

The poison theory has led to an over-working of the word

"pure", the idea being that an unprocessed food is pure because it has had no nasty chemicals added to it. In fact the reverse may be the case; the natural food may contain a poison that is removed in processing (natural cassava, for example, contains cyanide), and the impure food is often superior to the pure by virtue of the trace elements it contains. Two of the purest things in the kitchen cupboard are white sugar and table salt, both condemned by doctors and cranks alike as items to be avoided. So we can see that natural may not mean pure, and pure may not mean good.

The deficiency idea has developed from its original concept of a simple lack to a theory of balance. Certain nutrients need other nutrients to make them work, and substance A may be fairly useless without substance B to aid in its absorption, substance C to help it break down or substance D to prevent it breaking down too soon. Another aspect of balance is concentration. Take something out of a food and what is left may be too concentrated for the body to cope with. Many food reformers think concentration has more drastic effects than a straight lack of vitamins or minerals. Deficiencies are closely linked to food refining, factory farming and also to the simple mechanics of transport, storage and cooking. But according to some theorists, modern farming practice has given us another source of deficiency—the soil itself.

But before we go any further into the theories, let's have a quick look at what nutrition is all about. What makes us tick?

Dialogue

Q. *People who don't bother about their diet seem just as healthy as those who do. Why?*
A. Perhaps the operative word is "seem." During World War II, men called up for the US forces were found to be unfit in 50 per cent of the cases. These were men between eighteen and forty-five, so what about older people? Again, in Korea and Vietnam, autopsies on soldiers killed revealed a high propor-

tion of artery desease, yet they had been passed as fit when medically examined. It seems logical to assume that the results of wrong eating build up gradually over the years, so many young people who appear to be healthy now may be heading for trouble later on. Those who ridicule the idea that there is anything wrong with our diet point to the fact that our athletes are doing quite well on it. But athletes are young, and you cannot vindicate a diet by using young people as examples. Only if the middle-aged and elderly are fit does it prove anything. (See Chapter V.)

Q. *Surely we are in better health now than say a hundred years ago. Otherwise how could the population increase have come about?*
A. We are very much better off as regards bacterial and virus diseases because modern drugs have largely overcome these. Infant mortality has been greatly reduced, hence the population growth. But though the expectation of life has risen (fewer people die young), the average life span has not. This is because degenerative diseases have replaced infective and parasitic diseases as killers.

Q. *Is this not because diagnosis is better, or because more people are living longer so there are more degenerative diseases?*
A. Up to a point, yes, but statistics show that the so-called old age diseases, such as heart disease, are now occurring in younger age groups.

Q. *If our general health is declining from middle age on, cannot this be due to other things than food, such as stress and lack of exercise?*
A. Yes, it is generally agreed that all these things play a part, together with food.

Q. *Has the idea of auto-intoxication been definitely disproved?*

A. The laxative industry was founded on the idea that toxins could be re-absorbed from residues which remained too long in the digestive tract. The feelings of headache and malaise which went with constipation supported this idea. Then it was proved that the symptoms were caused not by poisons but by pressure on the nerve endings in the colon, and the idea of auto-intoxication went out of fashion for many years. Now, however, it is creeping back again, as recent researches described in Chapter V show.

Q. *Why do doctors on the whole discourage the idea that deficiences exist?*
A. For a variety of reasons, good and bad. On the bad side conservatism possibly, on the good side the desire to protect people from their own folly. Doctors are averse to self-diagnosis because they know how ignorant and gullible we are. "A little learning is a dangerous thing" and self-medication can cause trouble—for example vitamins A and D are toxic in excess. Though other vitamins can, as far as we know, be taken in any quantity, doctors say we are foolish to do so. Vitamins are effective in tiny doses, so the dictum "if a little is good, more is better" is nonsense. In the case of some minerals, it could be dangerous.

Then there is another aspect of self-diagnosis, one which lines the pockets of patent medicine manufacturers as well as supplement manufacturers. Many complaints have general symptoms such as lack of energy, irritability, aches and pains etc. Certain deficiencies may cause similar symptoms. So it is easy to conclude, if you feel sluggish and have a backache, that supplements will set you right. But since the symptoms may also mask more serious disease, self-diagnosis can be dangerous.

Q. *It seems as though there are two opposing groups—doctors and food reformers. Have they no common ground?*
A. It might be simpler to describe the two schools of thought as orthodox and unorthodox, for there are a number of qualified

doctors with distinctly unorthodox views, as we shall see in later chapters, and some surgeons who have become food reformers as a result of what they have seen in the course of their profession. But it is true to say that the two sides have little in common.

Q. *What about books putting forth the orthodox point of view?*
A. Probably the only orthodox scientist writing for a general rather than a specialist public is Dr. Magnus Pyke, author of *Man and Food, Teach Yourself Nutrition* and many others. Since he is not a food reformer, you have to go to the public library rather than the health food store for his books. They provide a very readable basis to the subject of nutrition, essential before embarking on more off-beat literature.

Q. *How does one pick out a reliable food reform book?*
A. It is very difficult for the non-scientist to know what makes sense and what doesn't. The danger with food reform books is that they are so persuasive. It is so easy to be won over by a well put case that one's powers of objective judgement (if any) are undermined. Here are some ideas for checking:

a.   Does the author contradict himself? You don't have to know the subject to spot a contradiction.
b.   Can you spot any mistakes? If something you chance to know about is wrong, perhaps things you don't know about are wrong too.
c.   Does the author know elementary chemistry? One food reform writer solemnly gives a list of foods containing carbon. (All foods contain carbon.) The same writer, in a later book, is indignant that the chemicals in fertilisers get into the crop. What else are they there for? Another writer, much given to public speaking, doesn't seem to know the difference between an atom and an electron. You don't have to be an expert to spot this sort of thing.
d.   Does the author know elementary arithmetic? It's

amazing how often, on checking a calculation, you find it doesn't add up.

e. Do the patients get cured rather too quickly? I suspect tales of old ladies, bedridden for years, who jump out of bed two days after eating some miracle food.

f. Is it up to date? Paperback best-sellers more than ten years old usually belong to the 'take lots of' school. They extol the virtues of the various nutrients but fail to mention the dangers of excess.

CHAPTER II

WHAT MAKES US TICK?

ONE OF THOSE wizards who specialises in startling statistics has worked out that half of all the chemical knowledge in history has been gained since 1950. That goes for organic chemistry, the chemistry of living matter, and includes the section which deals with nutrition.

Although the main principles of nutrition have been known for nearly two hundred years, the complexities are only just being unravelled now. Even the experts are groping in the dark, so it is not surprising that strange things happen when man tries to manipulate the chemistry he only partly understands.

The human body works on the same principle as a man-made machine, only far more efficiently. Fuel goes in, energy comes out. Energy comes from the combustion of fuel in both cases, but whereas the fuel of the machine is converted into work and heat, that of the living organism is converted into work, heat, growth and repair. Chemical reactions are constantly going on to this end, the whole process being termed metabolism. A child's guide to metabolism (as much as most of us want to cope with) goes something like this:

Food is our fuel, and the nutrients in food can be divided into five groups—proteins, carbohydrates, fats, vitamins and minerals. Why so many, and what do they do?

Carbohydrates (starches and sugars) and fats are energy foods, which when acted on by oxygen from the lungs are converted into energy, carbon dioxide and water. This is roughly what happens when coal burns. If more carbohydrate or fat is taken in than is needed for energy requirements, the surplus is stored in the form of body fat. As any weightwatcher knows, this is what dieting is all about. Carbohydrates consist of carbon, hydrogen and oxygen in varying proportions. During digestion they are split up and absorbed as glucose, or blood sugar. You could get sufficient glucose from starches without ever eating anything sweet. Examples of foods which are predominantly carbohydrate are cereals, sugar, honey, potatoes, root vegetables and bananas.

Fats (also carbon, hydrogen and oxygen) are often referred to as concentrated energy, because a given weight of fat produces more than twice as many calories as the same weight of carbohydrate or protein.

Proteins consist of carbon, hydrogen, oxygen and nitrogen with some minerals. These constituents are arranged in compounds called amino acids which are often referred to as building blocks, because they can be juggled around in different combinations to form body structures such as muscle, skin, hair, blood and so on. Proteins, together with minerals, are the growth and repair nutrients. Muscle protein, for example, is constantly breaking down and must be replaced. Protein can be oxidised to release energy also. If more protein is consumed than is needed, the surplus splits up; part becomes converted into fat while the nitrogen is eliminated mainly via the kidneys. Examples of protein-containing foods are meat, fish, eggs, cheese, milk, peas and beans.

How these groups of nutrients work together and the part they play in body metabolism is explained in more detail but very simply in Professor John Yudkin's book *This Slimming Business.* You don't have to be a dieter to enjoy it. The main thing to appreciate is that natural foods are mixtures of nutrients. For example, bread, which we regard as carbohydrate, contains 10-12 per cent protein and some fat. Milk consists of protein, fat and carbohydrate in fairly equal amounts. Only white sugar, an artificially produced food, is pure carbohydrate.

The body has often been likened to a chemical factory, but it is a factory with a difference. Whereas in a laboratory a process similar to digestion might require a whole day at very high temperatures, in the digestive tract it takes place in a few hours at a low temperature. This superior efficiency is achieved by enzymes. An enzyme is a catalyst, which, we may remember from school chemistry, is a substance which speeds up a reaction without taking part in it. Those busy statistical wizards tell us that although a mere thousand enzymes have been identified as yet, there are probably some five thousand in each human cell, and every minute throughout the body two million reactions requiring enzymes are taking place. An enzyme is a protein, with a minute amount of a mineral and/or vitamin included in it. Because the amounts are so small, the minerals in question are known as trace elements or trace minerals, and their action is only just beginning to be understood. The body can make its own enzymes provided the ingredients are present.

Triggering off basic reactions are the hormones, sometimes described as chemical messengers which stimulate action. Hormones are secreted direct into the bloodstream by endocrine or ductless glands, the most important of which are the pituitary (the master gland), thyroid, adrenals, pancreas and sex glands.

Minerals thus fall into two groups—the structural minerals, such as calcium and phosphorus which form bones and teeth, and the trace minerals already referred to as components of enzymes and hormones among other things. The minerals potassium and sodium exist as salts in the body fluids. Iron is needed for the red cells of the blood which carry oxygen. Lack of it causes anaemia. The best known of the trace minerals is iodine. Only a millionth of an ounce is needed daily, but a deficiency upsets the thyroid system which controls the metabolic rate, or pace of living.

Vitamins have been described as substances which are absolutely essential to health though only required in very small amounts. They cannot normally be made in the body but must be taken as food. Exceptions are vitamin D, which can be made by the action of sunlight on the oils of the skin, niacin, which can be synthesised from the amino acid tryptophan, and some other B vitamins which are synthesised by the intestinal bacteria. Some (possibly all) vitamins go in families or complexes. The vitamin B group consists of at least twelve members, the E group of eight and the K group of maybe ten. Those vitamins which are soluble in water (for example B and C) need to be taken every day. Those which are fat soluble (A, D, E and K) can be stored for several weeks.

What do vitamins do? A whole lot of different, unrelated jobs. For example, the B vitamins are co-enzymes, some involved in the metabolism of carbohydrates, and some with protein and fat. Vitamin C is concerned with the formation of connective tissue (the material between the cells), vitamin D with the absorption of calcium and phosphorus, vitamin K with blood clotting.

Before the nutrients can get to work on their various jobs, they have to be digested. Digestion starts in the mouth and continues in the stomach and small intestine, the components being split up by the enzymes in a series of digestive juices into forms which can dissolve in water. Some absorption takes place in the mouth and stomach but the main area of absorption is the small intestine which is surrounded by a network of blood-vessels which receive the nutrients. The bloodstream is the transport system which distributes the nutrients to the cells throughout the body. Oxygen, which we have seen is needed for the combustion process, is also carried to the cells by the blood.

That part of the food which is not required for metabolism, i.e. fibre, seeds and indigestible material, continues to the large intestine to be excreted.

Before it circulates through the body, the bloodstream from the small intestine passes to the liver where a sorting out process takes place. The liver is the main detoxicating organ, with the job (among others) of removing any poisons accidentally absorbed and sending them back to the intestines via the bile, a liver secretion which plays a part in digestion.

After the nutrients have been delivered to the cells and

oxidised, the by-products of metabolism, mainly carbon dioxide and water, are taken into the blood in exchange and conveyed to the organs of elimination. The carbon dioxide is given off by the lungs, together with some of the water. Surplus mineral salts and water are given off from the skin in the form of sweat. Other by-products, including the nitrogen compounds of protein metabolism, are eliminated via the kidneys. Since muscle protein is continually breaking down, these will appear in the urine, even if no protein is eaten.

So we can see that there are two "refuse disposal" systems in the body. The first gets rid of that part of food which cannot be digested—the faeces. The second gets rid of unwanted end-products of metabolism. To distinguish them, we can call the first excretion and the second elimination. The organs of elimination are the lungs, the kidneys and the skin.

So much for the child's guide. In actual fact it is a whole lot more complicated, since the chemical reactions releasing energy take place in a number of stages. This is how an expert puts it: "Fairly simple metabolites are 'burned' to form carbon dioxide and water with ATP as the high energy compound. An example of this is the system of dehydrogenating enzymes which pass reducing power to NAD, which, like succinate passes it on to the flavoprotein, which in turn passes it on to the essential metabolite ubiquinone and then on to oxygen via the cytochrome system. The process is called oxidative phosphorylation and is absolutely central in animal metabolism." Got it?

Luckily we don't have to be quite so erudite, but some expansion of the child's guide is necessary if we want to understand what food reformers are getting at when they talk about deficiencies and imbalances.

For instance, the metabolism of carbohydrate requires the assistance of some of the B vitamins. Vitamin B is soluble in water and therefore cannot be stored for long. If a refined carbohydrate is consumed, it may have had its vitamin B removed or greatly reduced. So either the temporary store has to be drawn on, causing a deficiency, or the chemical reaction has to stop half way for lack of sufficient vitamin B to complete it. The half-way stage involves a substance called pyruvic acid which is said to irritate the nerves. So, according to food reformers, people slightly deficient in vitamin B are nervous, irritable, have aches and pains and possibly even heart trouble owing to irritation of the nerves supplying the heart muscle. Severe deficiency causes definite diseases (see Chapter VI). Refined foods which lack sufficient vitamin B are white sugar (none), white rice (very little) and pre-war white flour. Since World War II, white flour in Britain and the USA has been enriched by restoring a portion of the B complex.

We have seen that proteins consist of amino acids. There are around thirty, some of which can be manufactured in the body and some of which cannot. Those which cannot (eight in number) are called essential amino acids because they have to be provided by food. Not all protein foods contain all the essential amino acids or contain them in the right quantities. Those which have them all (eggs come top of the class) are termed complete proteins, while those which lack some (mainly vegetable proteins) are referred to as incomplete. This is not as important as it sounds because with a mixed diet the deficiency in one food can be made good from another, as long as all are eaten at the same meal. (Officially, the terms complete and incomplete have been replaced by a series of "biological values".)

Proteins, as we have seen, are used for body building, but since the body's first priority is always for energy, protein would be converted to energy if it was the sole nutrient and repair would stop. This is somewhat hypothetical since no one normally tries to live on protein alone. The explorer Stefansson, while living with the Eskimos, made the mistake of trying to cut out fat and as a result became ill. Only when he restored fat to his diet did he recover.

The fat story is rather more complicated than appears at first sight, for it involves an extraordinary paradox. Fats are of two kinds—saturated or energy fats, and unsaturated or structural fats. The saturated fats, like carbohydrates, can be oxidised to release energy. The unsaturated fats are more like proteins in function—they are used in building cell membranes, arteries, nerves and brain. In fact it is very important that they should not be oxidised at all. If they are, not only are these structural materials destroyed but by-products are formed which are positively injurious, causing cell damage. Some theories suggest that this destructive process is the basis of ageing, and if it could be prevented, life could be prolonged. The paradox therefore, is that although life depends on oxidation, only the right substances must be oxidised; if the wrong substances are oxidised, the body destroys itself. A pretty problem you might think, but fortunately, in their natural state, the structural fats are protected by an anti-oxidant—vitamin E.

The simplest structural fats from which more complex forms can be built up have to be provided in the diet. For this reason they are known as essential fatty acids or EFA.

Unsaturated fats (including EFA) have a low melting point; they are usually liquid at room temperature whereas saturated fats are solid.

In recent years the idea that unsaturated fats are beneficial to heart cases has gained ground. This has led to a rush for the salad oil bottle and a craze for "soft" margarines which are not completely saturated. How fats are thought to be involved with heart disease is discussed in Chapter V.

We mentioned the action of hormones which, when released into the bloodstream, trigger off various physiological reactions. The stimulus which releases the hormone may be either chemical or mental, and misuse of this mechanism may have unforeseen effects. For example, chemical (or diet) stimulants acting via the hormone adrenalin include tea, coffee and cola drinks (all containing caffeine), cigarettes (nicotine), alcohol and strong condiments.

Among mental stimulants in primitive man were fear and anger, both requiring violent physical action—the fight or flight reaction. To these we now add the modern stress factors of frustration and tension. All these factors have the effect of boosting metabolism so as to mobilise the energy resources—extra sugar, fat and cholesterol are released into the bloodstream, the blood pressure goes slightly up to propel nutrients faster, the kidneys clear the bloodstream of wastes, and the decks are cleared for action. This is why we feel full of zest after tea or coffee.

But if the extra sugar is not converted into energy for physical action, it has to be taken out of the bloodstream again. Sometimes too much is taken out, so you soon need another boost. This is why people who drink endless cups of tea or coffee to keep them going, come to depend on it. Unfortunately cholesterol, once in the bloodstream, is not automatically removed; there is no special mechanism for it as there is with sugar. So it becomes a problem which increases with every traffic jam, delayed promotion, cancelled contract and unbeatable deadline in modern life.

A few generations ago, most tonics contained alcohol. Many still contain caffeine. But with the stress syndrome increasing daily, food reformers are coming to the conclusion that frequent stimulants rank next to poisons as items best avoided.

Knowing what makes you tick doesn't necessarily help you decide what foods to buy. We are told we have never been better fed. What, then, are the faddists complaining about? Their story is that the very things which appear to improve our food are in fact reducing its nutritional value. The marvels of science give with one hand and take away with the other. Processing and preservation remove vital nutrients, add poisons, affect balance and generally throw a monkey wrench in the works.

This is, of course, hotly denied by orthodox nutritionists, and while the battle rages, the harassed working housewife welcomes the growing supply of convenience foods. Those of us who would like to know more look hopefully round for an oracle. But who do we ask? Who, in fact, are the experts?

DIALOGUE

Q. *Dieters often try to do without carbohydrates or fats altogether. Is this possible?*

A. No. Nutritionists insist that all the food groups are essential. Where they disagree is on the ideal proportions of each. Proteins are the most obvious essential because they are needed for growth and repair. Since they slightly speed metabolism, they help the dieter to some extent. Carbohydrates are essential for energy and because sugar is the only nutrient used by the brain. Fat is essential owing to its slow action which allows gradual digestion of a meal. Without fat, you feel hungry again too soon. And, as we have seen, the unsaturated fats also act as building materials.

If you tried to live on protein alone you would suffer, oddly enough, from protein deficiency, because the amino acids would be broken down to release energy instead of being used for building. The brain would obtain its sugar this way. Carbohydrate alone would give energy without maintenance. Fat alone, as well as being nauseating, would be equally disastrous, since fat needs sugar to help break it down; without sugar the metabolism of fat stops half way, leaving substances called ketones which are poisonous.

In practice none of these things happen because all natural foods are mixtures of nutrients. But an excess of any group leads to disease.

Q. *If sugar is so essential, how do Eskimos survive on meat and fat?*

A. In freshly killed meat there is glycogen, the sugar stored in muscles and liver as an energy reserve.

Q. *What proportion of the diet should be protein?*

A. This is not generally agreed on, but official estimates have been going gradually down over recent years. What is agreed on is that it is very difficult, on an adequate diet, for an adult to get too little. The phrase "take care of the calories and the protein will take care of itself'' will cheer those who dislike calculation. A report of recommended allowances issued recently in Great Britain suggests 10 per cent of total calories as sufficient protein for adults, more for children. This figure is arrived at by calculating the minimum to attain nitrogen balance (5-6 per cent) then doubling it to make sure of adequate vitamin B which only occurs with protein. Even poor countries get this amount, the only doubt being the biological value of the protein, which is usually obtained from cereals or pulses. Some authorities think the amount should be a lot less.

It is important to realise that requirements differ with age. Children need protein for growth, so their requirements are high. But experiments with rats have shown that optimum health and long life are obtained by giving high protein during the growth period then low protein for the rest of life.

Q. *How does one translate the percentage into actual food?*
A. Ten per cent of total calories would come to between 220 and 280 calories. Since roughly four calories are produced from one gram of protein, this means between 55 and 70 grams (2-2½ ounces) of protein per day. We have to remember that an ounce of protein is not the same as an ounce of protein-containing food. Cheese contains 25 per cent protein, soya 40 per cent, meat, bread and other sources much less. A rough average of all sources is generally put at a sixth. So to get 2 ounces of protein you eat 12 ounces of protein food. This is all very interesting, but there's no need to take a slide rule to the table. Taking care of the calories will more than take care of the minimum. It may be the maximum we have to worry about in affluent countries. More about this in Chapters III and VIII.

Q. *What does biological value mean?*
A. A protein is complete if it contains all the essential amino acids. Those which have them in the correct proportions have the highest biological value. So, though there are many complete proteins they are not all of the same biological value. Recent research claims that there are more complete vegetable

proteins than was originally thought, and that uncooked protein has a higher biological value than cooked.

Q. *What proportion of the diet should be fat?*
A. Recommendations vary between 5 per cent and 35 per cent. Americans take 50 per cent of their calories as fat while the figure in Italy is put at 20 per cent and that for Japan at only 8 per cent. The proportion consumed in Britain has increased from 33 per cent in 1948 to approaching 50 per cent today. The danger mark is said to be 40 per cent but a lot depends on how much of the total is saturated. It is now recommended that at least a third of the fat intake should be unsaturated.

Q. *Why are fats sometimes called fatty acids?*
A. The word fat refers to a food (butter, suet, lard), the word fatty acid to a chemical component. Most fats consist of glycerol combined with three fatty acids. A fatty acid consists of a chain of carbon atoms each (except for the end ones) capable of combining with two hydrogen atoms. If all the carbon atoms in the chain have so combined, the fatty acid is said to be saturated, i.e. it has no room for taking on any more. If two adjacent carbon atoms have one, instead of two, hydrogen atoms attached, they become doubly bound to each other. A fatty acid with one such double bond is called monounsaturated; one with two or more double bonds is called polyunsaturated (PUFA). Like unattached girls at a dance, these carbon atoms are only too keen to find partners and unless protected by a chaperone (vitamin E) they are fair game for any stray oxygen atoms that come along. The fat is then rancid. Filling up the vacancies with hydrogen atoms turns the unsaturated fatty acid (liquid) into a saturated one (solid). The invention of hydrogenation at the beginning of the century meant that vegetable oils could be solidified to make margarine. Before this, margarine was made from animal fat. "Soft" margarine is only partly hydrogenated, leaving some PUFA.

There are many different fatty acids in an edible fat or oil. Butter, for example, consists of about sixteen, of which most are saturated. Whether an edible fat is termed saturated or unsaturated depends on the proportions of saturated, monounsaturated and poly-unsaturated fatty acids in its make-up. Some of the poly-unsaturated fatty acids (PUFA) can be built up in the body from simple forms. Simple forms which are needed in the diet are called essential fatty acids (EFA). So we can see that an EFA is always a PUFA, but not vice versa.

The PUFAs are sometimes referred to as structural fats because they can combine with other substances to build or repair body structures in the same way as proteins do. One of the things they combine with is cholesterol, a component of food which is also manufactured by the liver. By combining with cholesterol and preventing it from accumulating in the bloodstream, PUFAs help to prevent artery disease, hence the recommendation that a fair proportion of the fat intake should be PUFA.

Q. *Why do rats figure in so many nutrition experiments?*
A. Because like us they are omnivores, therefore they can be fed on the same foods as ourselves. Their life-span is conveniently short, ten days being roughly equivalent to a human year. Very few animals are omnivores, certainly no others so small, short-lived and convenient to keep. Guinea pigs, which are herbivores, are the only small mammals which do not make their own vitamin C, so they are used for experiments involving this vitamin.

Q. *What are the immediate results of a badly balanced diet?*
A. The results are fairly gradual. It has been said that there is only one disease—poor circulation. Since health depends on nutrients being carried to their destination by the bloodstream, any inadequacy in heart, blood vessels, capillaries and blood itself will be felt all over the body. With perfect circulation, there can be no disease. Since the bloodstream is protected by

the liver, which filters out undesirable components from the food, many people regard the liver as the basic organ, hence the saying "your liver is your life". Once impure blood is allowed to get past the liver and circulate (which happens when the liver is over-taxed) all sorts of diseases can result, depending on the nature of the "poison" which has got through. The elasticity of blood vessels and the viscosity of the blood become affected, blood circulates less efficiently, and deterioration sets in. Extremely sluggish circulation may even restrict oxygen supply to the brain, hence the mental confusion of some old people. So the priority seems to be a healthy liver.

Q. *Do liver salts keep the liver healthy?*
A. Millions of people must have been misled by the name "liver" salt into thinking so, but in fact the only direct action they have on the liver is to stimulate the flow of bile which helps digest fats. What the salts do is save the liver trouble by hurrying food through the digestive tract so that a portion of it never gets absorbed at all. This helps people who over-eat. Otherwise liver salts speed excretion by irritating the intestine and retaining water in the faeces. Though the salts are alkaline, they are too concentrated to act as an alkaline food.

So what is the best food for the liver? Alkaline salts! But not in the form of a laxative. Fruit and vegetables, a low-fat, medium-protein diet and plenty of exercise is the mixture recommended for liver health.

CHAPTER III

WHO ARE THE EXPERTS?

I N   1 9 6 9   a survey was run to find out what the average person knew about nutrition. Around 900 people were questioned, men and women, of all ages and incomes, and the results were published in a booklet entitled *Food Facts and Fallacies.* Of the 26 per cent who said they had gone to their doctor for advice on nutrition, only 2 per cent claimed to have learned anything. The evaluator remarks sadly, "In view of the almost complete absence of nutrition teaching in our medical schools there may be no discrepancy between these two figures. As the doctor is the one scientist in direct contact with the public, his lack of knowledge of the nutritional sciences is a serious gap in preventive medicine."

That incredible state of affairs is only just beginning to be rectified. But the gap, greater than any generation gap, for the time being remains.

We have to realise, with something of a shock, that doctors are only interested in disease, not health. They are trained to cure sickness, not to prevent it. (Naturopaths say the doctor doesn't cure you at all, you cure yourself.) Secondly, the doctor is not infallible. Far from being a superman, he is a human being like the rest of us, liable to make mistakes. Like the rest of us too, he values what little spare time he has; he likes to put his feet up rather than check up on all the latest research. After a twelve-hour day, with a night call in the offing, wouldn't you?

No, we can't really blame the doctor for the gap, any more than we can blame him for prescribing the pill and the tablet rather than a lecture on healthy living, because that is all there's time for and that is what the patient wants. Maybe it's an atavistic throw-back to the days of witchcraft, but most of us prefer a bottle of pills to a pep talk.

We have used the word doctor, so far, to describe the man with a brass plate outside his house. But there are countless others who *are* concerned with nutrition, very much so, and these are the research workers, doctors of another kind. They may be medically qualified or they may be bio-chemists or physiologists, but they are the people who discover new reactions, advance new theories and provide the basis on which food reformers work.

Between research workers and the public is a gap which could never be crossed without the help of middlemen, go-betweens or interpreters. They are people with sufficient brains to understand the research (though they are not cut out to do it) and to interpret the results. They paraphrase the learned papers of the scientists and give us the findings in language we can understand. They may have no degrees so scientists and doctors alike mistrust them. But where would we be without them? The first of a long line of middlemen was Gayelord Hauser. Now there are so many that we don't even remember their names.

There is a danger, of course, that the middleman may be a mere sensation seeker. The more superlatives he uses, the more miracle cures he describes, the better his book will sell. Because it is sometimes difficult to tell which category a writer comes into, the careful doctor condemns the lot, and possibly throws out the baby with the bathwater.

Very occasionally a scientist, like Professor John Yudkin, author of *This Slimming Business* and *Pure, White and Deadly,* decides to step into the limelight and be his own middleman. Provided he has the gift of writing simply, this is the best solution of all. But it is rare; mostly the backroom boys prefer obscurity.

So who are the advocates of food reform? The GPs, as we have seen, are against it (though they don't know much about it) while scientists are probably for it, to a limited extent. But their interest is restricted to the particular aspect they are working on. Mention Health Food to a research scientist and his reaction will be just as acid as that of the family doctor. So if doctors are happy with the present set-up, where did the voice of criticism come from?

It may come as a surprise to learn that the movement is far from new. The first beginnings were over a hundred years ago. What is new is the spread of interest and a public urge to know more about it. It is only recently that health food stores have sprung up in every town and health food manufacturing has become big business. Let's have a look at some of the main theories.

Nature Cure

Did you, like me, think Nature Cure was something gypsies did with herbs under the moon? Did you think that raw foods and juices were strictly for meditators and eccentrics and a spa was a place where retired colonels dipped their gouty toes into evil-smelling waters? On the contrary, Nature Cure is a perfectly sane, scientific idea. The theory, very briefly, is this: (1) we eat too much; (2) we eat too much protein and starch as opposed to fruit and vegetables, so cell metabolism is impeded and poisons accumulate; (3) all diseases, from head colds to fevers, are simply signs that the body is trying to rid itself of these poisons; (4) drugs, as prescribed by doctors, only make matters worse by curing the symptoms rather than the disease; the treatment is fasting, followed by juices, fruit, and a gradual return to a normal diet, normal in this case consisting of two to three times as much fruit and veg as other food. This proportion is based on the theory that primitive man was largely a fruit eater so the omnivorous diet must have been balanced roughly this way.

The "Father of Nature Cure" is said to be Vincent Priessnitz, a German who lived during the first half of the last century, at a time when doctors were relying increasingly on drugs. His cures were founded on simple diet, fresh air and exercise and the dictum "Nature heals", instead of doctor or medicine getting the credit. He also established the water cure (hydropathy) by which poisons are brought out of the system by means of compresses or baths. The patient is wrapped in wet sheets or a plastic cocoon, on the grounds that the skin is the largest and most neglected organ of elimination, and you can get a lot of poison out that way if you try.

Priessnitz had many followers in Germany and Austria during the second half of the nineteenth century and his ideas and methods also spread to the United States where schools and sanatoria were established. In England, several orthodox medical men became converted to the Nature Cure system with its anti-drug basis—the idea that while drugs can help an acute disease, they "go underground" and lead to worse troubles later on.

An interesting factor in this early history is that a number of the pioneers became converts through personal experience. Thus Priessnitz himself was helped to recover from an accident by means of water treatment, Louis Kuhne was "a physical wreck" until he discovered Nature Cure and made it his life work. Dr. James Jackson of the USA was given up as incurable by orthodox medicine at thirty-five, but lived to eighty-five after a year at a water cure establishment. Dr Henry Lindlahr, we are told, practised medicine until his own health failed. Then, finding his former skills useless, he turned to natural healing.

Food reform in Britain began early in this century, influence coming partly from Europe and partly from America. It is interesting to note that a Food Reform Restaurant, a health store and a Food Vitamin Café (what vitamins did they know about then?) were opened in London before World War I. However, the war prevented further activity until later. Also early in this century Dr Bircher-Benner opened his clinic in Zürich, and he is regarded by many as the founder of the health food movement as practised today. Though Dr Bircher-Benner's methods differ little from those of the early pioneers, he has sprung to fame in recent years partly owing to his daughter's book *(Eating Your Way to Health* by Ruth Bircher) and partly perhaps as the inventor of muesli, a granola-like cereal.

What is the difference between naturopathy and orthodox medicine? The fundamental difference lies in the two opposing theories of the cause of disease. Orthodox medicine believes that infectious diseases are caused by germs which arrive by accident. Naturopathy believes that disease is caused by a chemical imbalance (wrong eating) which has led to a build-up of poisons. It is the body's efforts to get rid of these poisons which give rise to the symptoms of the disease such as fever, catarrh or skin rash. The germs (which are of course present) are merely a by-product; only in a weakened system are they able to multiply.

These differences naturally lead to differences in treatment. The medical practitioner aims to kill the germs by means of antibiotics. The naturopath aims to put the body chemistry right. Killing germs, he says, merely suppresses a symptom and drives the disease underground, to reappear later in some other form, together with symptoms caused by the drugs themselves.

The fanatical nature cure addict believes in leaving it all to nature and possibly dies for his belief. The common-sense naturopath admits that when it is a case of a race against time, antibiotics must be used to save life, though this is not a cure in itself. When the danger is past, the patient's body chemistry must be put right and the drug poisons removed.

In his book *Fringe Medicine,* Brian Inglis illustrates the theory very neatly when he likens germs to rioters in a city where law and order has broken down. Stopping the riot is top priority, but the results are transient unless the problems causing the riot are dealt with too.

It is interesting to note that the "back to nature" cry, starting in the last century, has coincided with the refining of food and the increasing use of medicinal drugs. These two things are blamed for most of our trouble, and because they work slowly and gradually they may produce no dramatic ill-effects at all, just a general lessening of well-being which, with our usual pessimism, we attribute to middle age. People who have had a number of minor ailments, treated by drugs, will be worse off than those who have merely been eating refined foods all their lives. Manual workers and those who take a lot of exercise will have sweated some of their poisons out. So we're not all in the same state. But the basic idea prevails.

It is important to remember that the poisons Nature Cure is talking about are in the cells—unwanted by-products of metabolism given off by lungs, kidneys and skin. So the way to fix things up is to first of all give them a chance to drain away (a picture with great appeal) then to make sure you don't put any more back. This is done first of all by fasting, then by eating the right foods, in the right proportions, in small quantities.

While the draining away business is going on, poisons which have been lurking in the cells for years come out into the blood stream and give you hell. But not to worry, this is temporary, and shows all is going well. The important thing is to be prepared for this temporary set-back and not to panic into giving up the treatment. Once back to normal the things to eat are natural foods, which means whole foods, since nature knows better than we do how the components should be balanced. Also, we should eat far more fruit and vegetables as opposed to concentrated foods like meat and bread. This provides vitamins and minerals and bulk and sorts out the acid/alkali balance. Most of the foods we eat to excess—meat, starch, tea and coffee—are acid-forming, and too much acid is—you guessed it—poison. Too much alkali could be poison too, but under present conditions it is very rarely seen.

Does this mean that Nature Cure advises a vegetarian diet? Not necessarily. The two ideologies have much in common but they are not identical. In fact some naturopaths have no antipathy to meat in moderation. The main belief that binds all naturopaths is the belief in nature versus drugs, or even the need for drugs. In other words, eat right and you won't need treatment at all.

Vegetarians and Vegans
Far better known to the public than Nature Cure is vegetarian-ism, and at first sight the two seem to go together, for ''back to nature'' surely must mean nibbling a raw carrot in place of steak or roast beef.

Generally speaking, the two theories overlap but they are not the same. A naturopath recommends a diet roughly as follows: protein 10 per cent; fat 5 per cent; carbohydrate 20 per cent; fruit and vegetables 65 per cent. Some go further and put the last item at 70 per cent or more. The proteins don't have to be of vegetable origin though meat eating is discouraged on chemical rather than ethical grounds.

Vegetarians on the other hand are inclined to be more motivated by compassion, though they claim a scientific basis for their diet as well. The reasons often given for vegetarian-ism include the following:

1. Meat eating involves unnecessary killing. We can live perfectly healthily on vegetable proteins and, in fact, ''better health and longer life are more likely''. There have been many athletic records by vegetarians, far more in fact than one would expect from the proportion of vegetarian to meat-eating athletes. ''Athletes can clip those vital seconds to gain records by releasing their energy from dealing with toxic wastes associated with secondhand meat products.'' (By secondhand they mean food processed by an animal instead of direct from the source.)

2. Anatomically, man is more closely related to a vegetarian than a carnivore—long gut, grinding teeth, chewing jaws.

3. Meat eating is uneconomic. Land which will produce one ton of beef will produce ten to twenty tons of vegetable food. It takes 1.63 acres of land to feed a flesh eater as opposed to half an acre for a vegetarian. The world total of fertile land is about one acre per person, so the flesh eater is taking from somebody else. The present popula-tion of the world needs six million tons of protein a year,

but if this is animal protein, another hundred million tons of protein are needed for animal feed. This comes mainly from countries like India which need the food for their human population.

4. Meat eating is unhealthy. Meat not only contains growth-promoting antibiotics, synthetic hormones, vaccine residues, toxic wastes and bacteria, but the saturated animal fats which are thought to lead to heart disease. In Great Britain, those super-realists, the insurance companies, give better life policy rates to vegetarians and better cover to vegetarian restaurants in respect of food poisoning risks.

A vegan is a vegetarian who goes one step further and bans all animal products including milk and eggs, on ethical grounds. It is difficult to see at first how milking a cow involves cruelty, but vegans point out that the dairy farmer automatically kills all bull calves and the cow itself is slaughtered as soon as the milk yield ceases to be profitable. The same principle applies to poultry.

Vegans further point out that three-quarters of the earth's fertile land is used in feeding livestock, and though not as wasteful as meat, egg and milk products also require a disproportionate area of land for their production, and chickens and cows also eat imported grain. These are the environmental arguments. But there are health arguments too. Brucellosis, contracted from cow's milk, is on the increase. Unpasteurised milk can be dangerous, while pasteurised milk has lost much of its goodness. Finally, contamination by radio-active fallout is far greater in milk than in any vegetable food or commercial vegetable milk. These statements, say vegans, are supported by medical research.

The most commonly heard criticism of vegetarianism and veganism is that, with the exception of soya beans, no vegetable protein is complete. (See Chapter II.) However, this is not a serious snag as long as you mix your vegetables. Maize and beans, at one time the staple diet of some African tribes, add up to form a complete protein. So do many of the vegetables used in Chinese cooking. The sprinkling of cheese on minestrone soup is another example. The important thing is to get the right variety at one meal. Adding up over a period doesn't work. (Some nutritionists claim that many vegetable proteins have now been proved complete.)

A further criticism of veganism was that until recently the vitally important vitamin B12 was thought to occur·only in animal food. It is fairly well known (and often quoted by meat eaters) that Bernard Shaw suffered from anaemia and had to have liver injections to supplement his vegetarian diet. Possibly lack of B12 was his trouble. However, it has now been discovered that B12 is synthesised by bacteria which usually occur in the gut of animals but which may be found in soil or water contaminated by sewage. The bacteria can now be cultivated artificially in a vegetable medium and made to produce the vitamin without offending vegan feelings. There is also a claim that comfrey can absorb B12 from the soil, though this is not officially acknowledged.

The Meat Eaters

We have seen that the pioneers of Nature Cure in Europe had their disciples in the United States during the last century and that the movement there had some influence on those who introduced the new ideas to Britain. The whole cycle was to repeat itself, in a somewhat different way, when Gayelord Hauser started his fifty-year stint of activity in the nutrition field.

Gayelord Hauser tells us that as a boy he suffered from TB of the hip, was taken from Switzerland to the USA for treatment, and given up as incurable. Returning home to die, he was told by "an old man" (whether friend or medical adviser is not quite clear in the story) to eat only live foods, and after following this advice his troubles were over. "So eager was I to know more about the subject," he continues, "that I decided to make it my life's study."

At this time (the 1920s) there were in Europe a number of

diet centres, many though not all run on Nature Cure lines. Dr Bircher-Benner's Zurich clinic was flourishing, using a restricted diet instead of the fast usually advocated. The diet consisted of granola twice a day and lots of raw salad. The maxims "begin each meal with raw food" and "no day without green leaves" were followed. Meat was taboo.

There were other diets in vogue—grape cure, dry diet cure, and even a cure that involved meat three times a day. Hauser became a guinea pig and tried them all. He then summed up as his impression that all had one thing in common—an increase of elimination or a getting rid of poisons before building up the body on a "clean" foundation.

After this try-out of the clinics of Europe, Gayelord Hauser studied in America and became nutrition's best known middleman. That is, he sifted the findings of the research workers and interpreted them to the public. In the process he made his own judgements and developed his own answers which were passed on almost in the form of a crusade. In fact, sooner or later, all the best middlemen become crusaders. They not only interpret, they "do their own thing". So there were lectures and a school of dietetics in Chicago between the wars, then in the fifties a spate of books—*Diet Does It, Look Younger, Live Longer* and others. So the cycle—Europe, America, Britain —was repeated, but with the added impact of modern publicity media, so that the number of people who have at least heard of food reform is now far greater than it was the first time around.

Gayelord Hauser coined the expression "wonder food", eagerly seized upon by those looking for a short cut. His wonder foods were: brewer's yeast, yoghurt, wheat germ and molasses, all unheard-of, slightly gimmicky items at the time they were first introduced as sources of Vitamin B and other nutrients lost during refining. Now every health store sells them.

Gayelord Hauser is now in his late seventies and, according to the camera, still looks pretty handsome—the best possible advertisement for his diet. Another good-looking type, who started putting pen to paper some years later, is fellow American, Lelord Kordel, now in his late sixties. His general advice, similar to that of his forerunner, is set forth in the form of long cosy chats with imaginary patients. His wonder food is lecithin, needed to break down cholesterol, which is destroyed by refining or hydrogenation of oils (see Chapter VI). Since he believes strongly in the saturated fat theory of heart disease (see Chapter V) his writings are dotted with such slogans as "a doughnut is more deadly than a bullet".

These two crusaders have both turned manufacturer, producing respectively the Gayelord Hauser range of supplements and the Nutritime range, both extensively advertised in health magazines. Both writers are of interest, since they are high protein advocates and meat eaters, in contrast to followers of Nature Cure and the British school.

It is difficult, when told to eat "plenty of protein", to know how much plenty is, and many a woman's magazine must have set the dieter on to an egg-and-bacon—steak-or-chops—every-day regime (in the days when one could afford it). So it comes as a surprise to read in *The New Diet Does It* that protein should make up only 10-14 per cent of the diet: "over 18 per cent is positively harmful". In this Gayelord Hauser would receive the backing of most professional nutritionists as well as naturopaths. But reducing diets ("cut down on sugar and starch") rarely mention any upper limit to protein consumption.

However, Lelord Kordel and Adelle Davis appear to set no such limit. They say "have lots of protein", preferably in animal form. This, they think, gives them the stamina to get through a heavy day's work. Thus we find Kordel, with a lecturing programme ahead of him, ordering two chops for breakfast (barbaric, said the ladies at the next table), and Adelle Davis, in a similar position, opting for a hearty protein breakfast, fortified milk drinks hourly between lectures, and lobster for lunch.

Of the meat eaters, Gayelord Hauser, who sampled many nature cure regimes, is most tolerant of vegetarianism. He allows that the form in which you take your proteins is a matter of choice. Adelle Davis points out that the vegetarian must know something about nutrition if he is to do his adding up (of incomplete to complete proteins) successfully. But Lelord Kordel has no such inihibitons; he is convinced that most vegetarians are heading for trouble.

Describing an eight month experiment he did on himself, he declares that a reduced protein intake of "only one medium portion of cheese, egg, meat, fish or poultry a day" leads to exhaustion. Yet this is the amount a naturopath would regard as more than enough, provided one has a good mixture of vegetables and whole grain cereals. When he got back to three high protein meals a day, Kordel began to perk up, quite the reverse of what vegetarians would have us believe. Just give meatless meals a try, they say, and you'll never want to change back.

Who are we to believe? Perhaps the answer is "it's all in the mind"—you feel better when you expect to, or when some high powered crusader tells you you're going to. Or there may be another explanation—racial origin. People from northern latitudes, we are told, may be more adapted to meat eating than those from the sunny south, so one man's meat is literally another man's poison. More about this in the next chapter. Since both British and Americans are of mixed origin, it could be that we consist of different chemical types.

Despite the differences between the most vocal American nutritionists and the British on the subject of animal protein and amounts of protein in general, it is clear that what they have in common far outweighs the differences. What they agree on is deficiencies. Something is missing from our food which is causing most of today's health troubles. Epidemics have been vanquished but diseases of civilisation are on the increase. Because these diseases coincide largely with the refining of food, the increase in convenience foods, and with factory farming, the cry is "back to nature", back to whole foods, or some would say, health foods. But before we investigate the case for health foods, let's take a look at nutrition in the light of history.

DIALOGUE

Q. *If diet can cure disease, why are antibiotics used in an emergency?*
A. Because with an infectious disease (as opposed to a degenerative disease) diet cannot work fast enough. Bacteria multiply rapidly, producing their own toxins to add to the toxins causing the disease. Once a house has caught fire, you have to put the fire out before rebuilding with fire-proof materials. According to Nature Cure, orthodox medicine neglects the rebuilding part.

Q. *Are any types of food reform approved by doctors who do not have leanings towards Nature Cure?*
A. Quite a few approve the whole-food theory, the simplest and least cranky system, which overlaps many of the others. But there is strong official opposition to food reform in general, particularly theories supported by unqualified people. In July 1974, a whole supplement to *Nutrition Reviews,* issued by the American Nutrition Foundation, was devoted to showing up the alleged follies of a number of diets. Entitled "Nutrition Misinformation and Food Faddism", the review gives short shrift to Adelle Davis, Dr Linus Pauling, macrobiotics, organic farming, vitamin therapy, veganism and several other lesser known diets. The Food and Drug Administration is introducing some anti-health-food regulations which prohibit claims that, (1) natural vitamins are superior to synthetic; (2) organic produce is nutritionally superior; (3) vitamin P and lesser B vitamins are of nutritive value, and (4) that transport, storage and cooking of foods may affect value—a somewhat puzzling item. Also, there is a strong move to tighten up on definitions of health foods.

Q. *What is osteopathy? What is chiropractice?*
A. Osteopathy is a lot more than fixing dislocated joints. An osteopath works on the theory that many ailments can be traced to faulty anatomy such as pressure on nerves emerging from the spinal column. This may even affect digestion and other functions. Hence the cure by manipulation. Chiropractice is a stage of osteopathy; the chiropractor concentrates on the spine alone, the osteopath studies the whole body. They have no direct interest in diet though the osteopath works closely with the naturopath at a health farm.

Q. *What is macrobiotics?*
A. This is a dietary system which appeals to those who like a touch of oriental mystery in their lives. Publicised by Dr George Osawa, it hails from Japan and includes so many exotic bits and pieces in the recipes that enthusiasts unable to track down all the ingredients find themselves close to starvation. As a result, those who have been over-eating suddenly feel much better but those who were eating normally start to fade away. Shorn of all the mumbo-jumbo, the diet is a simple attempt to balance opposites (usually acid and alkali but not always) called yin and yang. If you read the small print which advises sticking to foods grown within five hundred miles of home, you find yourself with an ordinary natural diet. But this means goodbye to brown rice and the glamour of the east.

It is said by some naturopaths that the word macrobiotic (which is of Greek origin anyway) was used many years ago to apply to a diet for health and long life. But this was quite a different system from the present popular cult of that name.

Q. *Is there any scientific proof that a vegetarian diet is healthier?*
A. Some say the advantage of a vegetarian diet lies not so much in the absence of meat as in the presence of vegetables—we do not normally eat enough of them. Since vegetarians eat bread, potatoes and sugar, they are just as liable to be over-weight as anybody else, unless they follow the 3:1 ratio of

vegetables to concentrates. A recent study of twenty-two elderly vegetarians showed that they had above average levels of vitamins B1, B2 and C and none of the tongue and skin disorders so often seen in elderly people as a result of deficiency. The report concludes cautiously: "It is not possible to say on this evidence alone that the absence of the signs in twenty-two vegetarians was attributable to high vitamin intake."

Q. *What is the case against excess protein?*
A. All surplus protein (vegetable as well as animal) leaves a residue which contains the nitrogen fraction. Normally this is eliminated by the kidneys as urea, but habitual excess puts a strain on the kidneys which may eventually damage them so that they function less efficiently. Some forms of protein also form uric acid. Uric acid not eliminated circulates in the blood causing possible artery damage and rheumatic troubles. Many people think that hardening of the arteries is caused by urate deposits from excess protein.

Proteins are mild stimulants (hence the meat feast by warring tribes before a battle); they increase the metabolic rate, which is why you feel the need for more protein in cold weather. But too much can overtax the system. Though protein aids calcium absorption, too much causes excretion and osteoporosis may result.

Q. *What is the case against meat in particular?*
A. When an animal is killed and blood ceases to flow, the composition of the muscle changes providing a medium for bacteria. So any meat eater has to cope with a certain amount of poison as a by-product. Carnivores get over this problem by having a short gut for rapid excretion and a large liver to deal with the poisons produced by the bacteria. But human anatomy is not really suited to a meat diet, say vegetarians.

Orthodox nutritionists say meat is no more toxic than any other protein. The middle of the road view is that we can cope with meat in moderation. Exercise, which speeds the passage of residue through the gut, helps. Primitive man with his active life was better adapted to meat eating than we are today. It is generally agreed that the idea of meat as an essential for strength and athletic performance is now outmoded. Any protein of similar biological value is equally good.

Q. *If a fairly low protein diet for adults is generally agreed upon, where did the idea of high protein come from?*
A.   1. Probably from requirements originally. If you tell people to cut starch and sugar, you have to provide a substitute to cheer them up. Most food reformers would recommend fruit and vegetables as the substitute, but this has never been official policy, and protein has hitherto been considered beneficial in any quantity.

2. Then there is a theory that people under stress need a lot of protein. Lelord Kordel suggests that we actually use up 40-60 grams a day (the whole allowance according to recent estimates) when under stress. The high protein diet advocated by several American nutritionists is based to some extent on stress requirements.

3. The stimulating effect of protein which results in a feeling of warmth and well-being, so that one associates protein with strength.

4. The fact that protein (and its associated fat) are low satiety foods, slowly absorbed and long-lasting in contrast to carbohydrate. If you want to keep going for several hours without a snack, protein is what you need. The only question is, how much?

CHAPTER IV

BACK TO BASICS

W I T H   E C O L O G Y (the relationship between living creatures and their environment) now the in thing, nutritionists of
all creeds are getting interested in evolution. What sort of food
did the first human beings have, and how have we evolved and
adapted to changing conditions since then?

There seem to be two opposing theories as to how we
started. One, based on the discoveries of early man in Africa,
which show him as an armed predator, using weapons in place
of claws and teeth, assumes our ancestors were almost entirely
carnivorous. The other prefers the idea that our common
ancestry with apes kept us vegetarians for much longer and
that it was only during the ice age that man was forced to turn
meat eater. "Eskimos living entirely on flesh and our own
butchers' shops, are unhappy remnants of those catastrophic
times," says one vegetarian pamphlet.

However, our anatomy seems to point to an omnivorous
diet. The digestive tract is longer than that of a carnivore,
shorter than that of a herbivore. We have canine teeth of a sort:
incisors for dealing with meat and molars for grinding. Our
jaws move sideways (herbivore) as well as up and down
(carnivore). But we do not need to chew as much as the apes
with their heavy jaws and jaw muscles which have to be
attached to the top of the head. We have alkaline saliva for
dealing with starches whereas carnivores have acid saliva for
dealing with meat.

In spite of all this there is some disagreement on what
proportion of meat and vegetables an omnivore needs. Some

say, "Primitive man subsisted on a diet of fruits, berries and nuts primarily, with animal additives of insects and eggs and small birds when he could catch them". This ignores the weapons found with the early fossils which must have been used for something more challenging than small birds. Others suggest that the diet was "mostly meat and offal with occasionally vegetable foods such as leaves, fruit, berries and roots". Perhaps the most generally accepted theory is that early man was a hunter-gatherer, catching what prey he could with his weapons and filling up with specially collected fruits and vegetables.

The main difference between this diet and our present one is that there were no concentrated cereals or carbohydrates—no flour, no bread and no sugar as we know it. It was only about ten thousand years ago—very recently in evolutionary time—that agriculture started, developing cereals in a big way and providing the flour products which now we should feel lost without. Before this, carbohydrates came from fruits and roots and formed a comparatively small part of the diet. Secondly, the replacement of hunting by animal husbandry made life less precarious. For most, these changes meant a settled life though there were (and still are) some people who preferred to wander with their flocks and herds, living almost entirely on animal foods.

Evolution comes from the adaptation of a species to its environment, so that any change in the organism which benefits the species, tends to survive. Scientists tell us that adaptations to changes in the environment take a long time to evolve, and from somewhere has come the figure thirty thousand years. This means that we have not yet had time to adapt physiologically to any change that took place less than thirty thousand years ago. So agriculture, with its resulting increase in carbohydrate consumption, is too new for our systems to have caught up with, and it is the diet of the hunter-gatherer, with its low carbohydrate, which our bodies really need.

This theory, which is by no means supported by all, pleases both vegetarians and high protein advocates, for both unite in condemning the excess carbohydrate consumption of modern man, particularly the refined kind we eat today.

As the human race spread from its tropical Garden of Eden to the less hospitable climate of the north, less vegetable matter was available so the meat component of the diet increased. Thus we have at one extreme the arctic Eskimos, who until recently lived entirely on meat and fish, and at the other those tropical people in Africa and Asia who are entirely vegetarian. The theory makes sense though it does not account for those tropical tribes of wandering pastoralists who live on milk, blood and some meat, but no vegetables. However, it accounts for the fact that we are not all chemically the same, and suggests that the battle between meat-eaters and vegetarians may be resolved by admitting their ancestral differences.

Another aspect of the primitive diet which appeals to food reformers is that it was balanced by nature. We ate what was good for us in the right proportions because we had become adapted to benefit from what was available, and instinct told us what to eat. The reason instinct guides us no longer is that palatability and nutritive value have now become separated by technology (flavour can be artificially manufactured) so that something that appeals to the taste may be the very reverse of what we need. As tampering with food becomes the rule rather than the exception, natural balance is upset.

Using the evolutionary approach, these are the ways in which food reformers think the modern diet falls short of the ideal:

1. It contains too much carbohydrate (particularly refined).
2. Far more bulk is needed, as this is what a primitive diet with its high vegetable intake would include. Bulk, as we know, prevents constipation, which, far from being the trivial matter most people think, can be the forerunner of far more serious things.

3. The modern diet is too acid, since both meat and cereals are acid-forming, while most fruits and vegetables leave an alkaline residue.

4. The modern diet is too low in vitamin C of which fruit and vegetables are the main source. Linus Pauling, Nobel Prize winner and author of *Vitamin C and the Common Cold,* is one of those who believe early man to have been mainly vegetarian. He attributes many of our ills to the fact that the comparatively low plant food intake of today gives us much less vitamin C than our ancestors would have had.

5. The modern diet is fragmented and therefore unbalanced. Early man ate the whole animal, including the organs; we eat mainly muscle meat. He ate the whole fish, including the bones, the whole fruit, including the skin, and whole grains, including germ and husk. Nutrients which may be missing from some parts of food are present in other parts, so that whole foods are the best sources of all required nutrients, including those 'which are still unknown.

6. The wild game eaten by early man contained much less saturated fat than domestic animals have, especially those raised under intensive farming methods. The balance between saturated and unsaturated fats was therefore much better.

The man whose name is most closely linked with the wholefood theory was, fortunately for the image of the food reform movement, a genuine doctor. He was Sir Robert McCarrison, Director of Nutrition Research in India during the 1920s and later Director of Postgraduate Medical Studies, Oxford. In the mountains of the extreme north-west of India, (now Pakistan) he came across a supremely healthy tribe—the Hunzas—who lived in a remote valley cut off from civilisation. Not only was disease unknown, but crime was practically non-existent too. There were no police, no prisons. Yet only a few miles away, in the part of India where refined foods were available, all the diseases of civilisation were present.

Until a few years ago, the only way into Hunza was on foot or horseback through a narrow river gorge. Then a jeep track was built and a small trickle of tourists was able to visit these unusual people. In 1970, when I visited Hunza, there were still no police and no prisons but one or two small shops had opened and currency, formerly non-existent, was in use. With Chinese aid a larger road, for normal traffic, was being built and the state was on the verge of being opened to the outside world.

Sir Robert McCarrison attributed the health of the people to their food which in turn depended on their method of farming. Crops are grown on narrow terraces cut out of the steep mountain side. Sometimes these are mere troughs cut in the rock, with soil and compost carried up. The larger terraces are supported by carefully built stone walls. Waters from the glaciers, rich in minerals, are diverted for irrigation. With this type of land, there is little space for livestock. A few goats and sheep are kept, mainly for milk and wool. Little meat is eaten but fruit forms a large part of the diet—apricots, mulberries, apples and grapes. It is apparently the composting that does the trick, enabling a small acreage to produce crops year after year without deterioration. I was interested to hear, in 1970, that the Pakistan Government had tried to persuade the Hunzas to use chemical fertilisers in order to increase yields, but this had been refused.

To see just how important diet was, Sir Robert McCarrison did some experiments which have since become classics, quoted in many books on nutrition. He fed groups of rats on (1) the diet of the Hunzas, (2) the white rice diet of the Indians of the south, and (3) the diet of the British working man. Group 1 flourished, Group 2 developed a variety of diseases and Group 3 became cannibals as well.

About the time McCarrison was working in Hunza and concluding that whole food was responsible for the people's health, an agriculturalist also in India was coming to similar conclusions by a different route. He was Sir Albert Howard, Imperial Chemical Botanist to the Government of India. His job was to find a method of increasing crop production by means that the peasant farmer could afford, which of course excluded chemical fertilisers. He devised a system of composting known as the Indore method. Crops grown on land treated by this method became resistant to disease, and this resistance was passed on to livestock fed on these crops to such an extent that oxen so fed could mix with oxen suffering from foot and mouth disease without becoming infected.

Back in England, Sir Robert McCarrison gave a number of lectures on his findings, and as might be expected, there was little reaction. But lest this book has given the impression that the only good doctor is a dead doctor, it must now be emphasised that the next step in the story was taken by medical men. In 1939 a group of general practitioners published a paper entitled "Medical Testament", in which they drew attention to McCarrison's experiments and went one step further. They suggested that there were other isolated communities who also enjoyed perfect health, namely the Eskimos and the islanders of Tristan de Cunha. The diets of these three groups differed drastically but what they had in common was that all were based on a natural system of agriculture, as advocated by ecology, in which animal and vegetable residues were returned to the soil (the "soil" in some cases being the sea). The two lines of investigation were thus linked together to form the basis of an entirely new approach to health via nutrition.

The Medical Testament ended: "We are called upon to cure sickness. We conceive it to be our duty in the present state of knowledge to point out that much, perhaps the most of this sickness is preventable and would be prevented by the right feeding of our people. We consider this opinion so important that this document is drawn up in an endeavour to express it and to make it public."

In 1940 experimental work was started to evaluate three

systems of farming from the health point of view. These were (1) an entirely natural system based on the ecological cycle, (2) an entirely artificial system based on chemical fertilisers and pesticides, and (3) a mixed system using manure supplemented by chemical fertilisers.

While the farming experiment was getting started, Lady Eve Balfour wrote her book *The Living Soil*. The theory which is explained in this book revolves round the word "living". The top few inches of any good soil contain a wriggling, squirming mass of living creatures ranging in size from bacteria to earthworms. Some are beneficial to plants, some are enemies; but a healthy plant is able to achieve a balance and to live in harmony with its environment, aided by the "good" worms, fungi and bacteria, which are absolutely essential to the whole life process. For this balance to continue, the living part of the soil, or humus, must be maintained.

Humus is derived from organic matter, such as plant residues and animal excrement, processed by bacteria to a form which the plant can utilise. The top soil is made up of soil particles interlaced with humus, air and water. In nature (as in a forest), humus is maintained automatically but very slowly. When crops are grown and taken away, humus must be renewed more rapidly by preparing it separately, in a form called compost, and spreading it on the fields. Compost can be made from anything which was once living—plant remains, manure, sawdust, egg shells, bones—plus soil to supply the bacteria and worms to start the ball rolling.

But why go to all this trouble when you can buy fertiliser by the bag? It is easy to see how the indiscriminate use of pesticides can poison soil and crops, but it is at first difficult to see how the use of artificial fertilisers can do harm. Remember those school botany experiments, when we grew plants in jars of water with different chemicals added? It all seemed quite logical, and to the vast majority it still does.

The chemical idea originated around 1840 when a German chemist named von Liebig analysed the ash remaining after plants were burned, and concluded that what he found (which was salts of nitrogen, phosphorus and potassium) was what plants took from the soil, and therefore all that need ever be put back. The idea caught on like magic and the fertiliser business was born.

According to the chemists, vast quantities of these salts are needed by crops, far more than can ever be supplied by compost. Compost is all very nice for your garden if it amuses you to make it, they imply, but it is quite inadequate for commercial farming. The organic school's reply to this is that the chemists have missed the whole point. It is not claimed that compost contains enough minerals for the plant's needs. What is claimed is that compost acts on the soil population, stimulating the bacteria, fungi and forms to produce the necessary nutrients in these ways:

1. Soil bacteria break down insoluble mineral salts slowly and make them available to the plant. (Bacteria are reduced by fertiliser.)
2. Soil fungi produce a substance which stimulates the root system of plants so that more nutrients can be absorbed. (Fungi are reduced by fertiliser.)
3. Certain plants have fungi growing inside their roots, to the benefit of both. This is known as the microrhizal association. Spectacular growth rates are shown by plants with microrhiza.
4. Earthworms (which are reduced by fertilisers) burrow five or six feet down, aerating the soil and releasing minerals locked in the subsoil.
5. The dead bodies of the soil population themselves provide a source of plant food, particularly nitrogen. Bodies of earthworms alone are said to add 1,000 lb of nitrogen fertiliser to each acre.

The case for compost therefore is that it supplies the necessary plant nutrients indirectly rather than directly, and by enabling earthworms to survive, it allows the soil to be aerated and a good soil structure to be maintained. The case against chemical fertilisers is:

1. They short-circuit the natural process. Being soluble in water, they form strong solutions which crowd out many other nutrients already in the soil (possibly trace minerals) and by being readily available cause a too rapid growth.
2. Substances added to the fertilisers to make them soluble are toxic to the soil population so that the functions mentioned above cannot be performed by them.
3. Plants grown with chemical fertilisers lose their resistance to disease. The reason is that some of the micro-organisms mentioned above protect the plant. For example there is a microrhizal fungus which actually digests eelworms (parasites). And earthworms, by their aerating activity, kill off dangerous bacteria which can only exist in the absence of air. Some moulds seem to act as plant antibiotics. All these are reduced by chemical fertilisers. Resistance to disease is vital in view of the possible dangers of insecticides and their high cost.
4. Fertilisers stimulate rapid growth giving high yields. But. cell walls are thin and water content high. Nutrients are diluted, lessening flavour and value. This may account for the greater susceptibility of such plants to disease and the fact that they do not keep so well.
5. Since fertilisers reduce bacteria, they reduce the amount of humus in the soil. When there is no humus, the water-retaining power of the soil is affected and it becomes easily eroded by wind or rain.
6. As humus is reduced, increasing amounts of fertiliser are needed to maintain yields, so the whole production cost escalates.

When *The Living Soil* was written, thirty years ago, enzymes were not so much in the public eye as they are now, and trace minerals came somewhere near the bottom of the scale as vital items of diet. Now, however, the importance of trace minerals as components of enzymes is appreciated and some of the rather spectacular results of composting, which cannot be explained otherwise, make sense in this context. There is evidence that trace minerals in the soil are made available to the plant by the action of bacteria in a more easily assimilable form than if they were associated with inorganic chemicals. Supporting this, it has been shown that the trace mineral content of grain has declined over the last few years.

The advantages of composting are therefore:
1. Preservation of soil structure and prevention of erosion.
2. Resistance of crops to disease.
3. Cheapness of materials as compared with fertilisers.

The disadvantages are:
1. Increased labour costs on farms without livestock.
2. Insufficient materials available.
3. High cost of transporting manure if needed from outside.

Supporters of organic farming claim that compost at the rate of 5 tons to the acre per year is adequate once soil fertility has been restored, and that one man can make sufficient compost for 100 acres per year. Materials would be available if household rubbish could be diverted for composting with sewage. A number of municipalities already make compost in this way and sell it.

To many who have not read the arguments in *The Living Soil,* the organic farming idea is so much muddle-headed moonshine. Elspeth Huxley, more charitable than most, describes the theory as a religion which you cannot argue about—"like all faiths, it operates on a different wavelength". This is due to bad public relations on the part of the organic folk, who tend to ramble on about vital forces, without explaining what they really mean.

The Living Soil has now been revised and reprinted, under the title *Story of the Haughley Experiment.*

After thirty years, has the nutritional superiority of organically grown produce been proved? From chemical analysis—no. But advocates of compost farming are pinning their hopes on something called micro-electric tension which is the subject of research at the moment. We know that minerals in the body fluids carry electric charges and that nerve impulses depend on this. We also have the theory that compost favours the intake of trace elements by the plant. So when all this is put together we may find that the connection between food and "vital forces" is not such a flight of fancy as we tend to think.

McCarrison and Howard did their pioneer work fifty years ago. Let us return to the present and view the diseases of civilisation in the light of modern research.

D I A L O G U E

Q. *Is there any evidence that primitive people were healthier and that their health was due to diet?*
A. No, only a supposition that they must have been tough to live the life they did. But the lifespan was short. Also, fossils have been found showing signs of rickets, so all was not perfect in the garden of Eden.

Q. *Is there any proof that our more recent ancestors were healthier?*
A. No, we have evidence that they were even less healthy but their diseases were different from those of today. With civilisation came overcrowding and the diseases due to unhygienic conditions. Man has not yet discovered the secret of how to live. In the past (as now) the rich, who could afford good food, ate too much and took too little exercise, while the poor had an unbalanced diet, or simply not enough. And, as we have seen, food deterioration was a big problem. Some enthusiasts assume that refining is the main evil, and that before refining

everyone was hale and hearty. But there have always been snags, mainly due to ignorance.

Q. *Is there any proof that organic produce affects health?*
A. Not human health. There is the evidence of Howard's work indicating that livestock fed on compost-grown crops were resistant to disease. More recently, there are claims that a map of the foot and mouth disease areas in Europe coincides with a map dividing commercial from peasant farming areas. The implication is that the peasants who still follow the old-fashioned methods have disease-resistant cattle. This being so, one could make a guess that humans eating compost-grown crops might also be resistant to disease, but it is pretty impossible to prove such a thing. Lady Eve Balfour claims that after ''going organic'' she said goodbye to rheumatism. And there are claims from certain schools, compost-growing their own vegetables, that the children improved in health. But the evidence is too vague to impress a scientist.

Q. *Is there any proof that whole foods are better for health?*
A. It all depends on what you mean by whole foods. A scientist who wanted to get rid of me enquired sarcastically, ''Do you mean that when we eat a carrot we should eat the top?'' You have to draw the line somewhere—even primitive man would not eat the shells of nuts, the hide of animals, or the feathers of birds. So, having been floored by the scientist, I now define whole food as something that cannot be split up by hand. An ape can peel a banana or take the top off a carrot, but it cannot take the germ out of wheat. In other words, whole foods are unrefined foods, with nothing added either. Are they better for health? More about this in Chapters V and VI.

But the whole-food argument does not rest entirely on the refining issue. There is the argument that wholefoods are ''balanced as in nature, in the right proportions''. What this means it is difficult to say, for the proportion of protein in wheat may be low and that in peanuts high, so what proportion you finally end up with depends on how much of each you eat—it has nothing in particular to do with wholeness.

Then there is the "Mother Nature in her wisdom . . ." school of thought, which implies that a benevolent nature has arranged the components of every edible plant for the sole benefit of man, with the necessary ingredients for metabolising it all wrapped up in one package. But this is not so at all. Quite often there are poisons wrapped up in the package, and man has to use his ingenuity to get rid of them. From the evolutionary standpoint the Mother Nature school have got things back to front. Nature does not provide a package deal; on the contrary, it is the species which adapts best to available food sources which comes out on top.

Q. If McCarrison's findings were so conclusive, why are they ignored by majority medical opinion?

A. Some people think they were not conclusive. The argument is that McCarrison was comparing good diets with bad diets rather than wholefoods, compost-grown, with processed foods. The Indians of the south, it is claimed, were simply undernourished. Their diet lacked essentials so it is not surprising that they (and the rats on the same diet) were stunted and sickly. The experiment proves the virtue of a balanced diet, not the superiority of wholefoods or compost-grown crops. But McCarrison had many sympathisers in the medical world, and his followers still work today to spread his ideas. It has been suggested that his findings came at the wrong time. During the 1930s, when his theories were going round, great strides were made in pharmaceutical research. The sulfa drugs, followed by the antibiotics, were discovered, with their miraculous powers of curing hitherto killer infectious diseases. They stole the limelight, and being quick-acting, had much greater appeal for doctor and patient alike than a mere diet theory. McCarrison's studies were overshadowed by the new therapy and forgotten during World War II.

CHAPTER V

DISEASES OF CIVILISATION

THE TERM "DISEASES of civilisation" is used to refer to those diseases which have increased dramatically during this century in affluent countries while remaining rare or unknown in primitive societies. They include:

1. Coronary heart disease, the No. 1 killer in the United States, Britain, and other so-called civilised countries, and strokes.
2. Diabetes, which now ranks third as a killer as against 27th place in 1900.
3. Ulcers.
4. Constipation and resulting maladies.
5. Mental troubles.
6. Cancer, the No. 2 killer but placed last because we will not be discussing it here.

These are degenerative non-infectious diseases, usually, though not always, affecting older people. They cannot be blamed on germs or parasites. So what is their cause?

While there is a reluctance on the part of the sceptical public to accept any theory put forward by unorthodox people (naturopaths, self-trained nutritionists or diet crusaders), when research workers and doctors get involved they command respect. There are a number of qualified people who are convinced that civilised, or degenerative, diseases can be laid at the door of civilised food. They have put pen to paper to tell us why, and if they disagree violently with each other, or reach the same conclusions by different routes, at least the reader is stimulated by their arguments to think for himself.

Recent publications on the subject of degenerative diseases include: *Diabetes, Coronary Thrombosis and the Saccharine Disease,* by T. L. Cleave, G. D. Campbell and N. S. Painter; *Pure, White and Deadly* by John Yudkin; *What We Eat Today* by M. A. Crawford; *Food Is Your Best Medicine* by H. G. Bieler; *Health Hazards of a Western Diet* by G. A. Stanton; *Some Diseases Characteristic of Modern Western Civilisation* by D. P. Burkitt; and *Natural Health, Sugar and the Criminal Mind* by J. I. Rodale.

The authors of the first book, which we can shorten for simplicity to *The Saccharine Disease,* claim that refined carbohydrates (not only sugar) are responsible for a variety of modern diseases, which because of their common cause, can be grouped together. The word "saccharine", they tell us, means "related to sugar" and should be pronounced to rhyme with Rhine; it has nothing to do with saccharin, the chemical sweetener, which is pronounced differently.

The book is based on the law of adaptation which requires the diet to consist of foods to which man has become adapted through evolution. But the authors do not support the view that the comparatively recent advent of agriculture, resulting in high carbohydrate intake, presents any problem in adaptation. They believe our ancestors were fruit-eaters and point out that there are many primitive societies today who live almost entirely on carbohydrates, without suffering any ill effects. It is the recent innovation of refining which they blame for much of today's ill-health. The refining of carbohydrates, they say, produces its effect on the body in three ways: (1) through concentration, which leads to over-consumption, (2) through the removal of fibre, (3) through the removal of protein.

1. *Concentration*
Refining makes it easy to eat too much without realising it. For example, the amount of sugar which one normally has with a pot of coffee is equivalent to six apples; the average daily intake of sugar is equivalent to two and a half pounds of sugar beet. In both cases, the natural product is self limiting, the

refined product is not. Similarly, wholemeal bread, containing bran, is much more difficult to eat in quantity than white bread. From this over-consumption we get the diseases of obesity, diabetes and coronary thrombosis.

Obesity may mask malnutrition, since stuffing oneself with too much carbohydrate can mean a crowding out of other necessary nutrients such as protein and minerals, so that a feeling of satiety can go hand in hand with deficiency. The natural balance has been upset.

The authors make the interesting point that there is no such thing as an overweight wild animal; if we stuck to unrefined carbohydrates, we should have no weight problems either. Lest unsuccessful dieters hail this idea as an answer to prayer, it must be pointed out that limiting one's carbohydrate to bran bread, preferably two days old, may not be everybody's idea of dieting without tears.

Over-consumption may also lead to the most common form of diabetes which appears in middle age. We know that insulin, secreted by the pancreas, is needed to convert glucose (blood sugar) into glycogen (the stored form), and that as blood sugar rises, during a meal, insulin production is stimulated. Refined sugar passes very rapidly into the bloodstream, requiring rapid action by the pancreas to deal with it. In time, this high rate of production causes the pancreas to break down.

Long before the pancreas actually gives up, it causes trouble by over-reacting. In response to high sugar intake, it actually secretes more insulin than necessary, so that the blood sugar level drops below normal. The subject then suffers from hypoglycaemia or low blood sugar. He feels weak, takes more sugar to pull himself together, and so a vicious cycle is set up, the body acting rather like a learner driver who over-corrects the steering until he finally crashes into the ditch. This over-correcting may continue for years before disaster strikes, and if only it was understood, the final outcome of diabetes might be avoided. The diabetic needs regular medication to keep him alive. The disease is now so common that special diabetic jams are available in the supermarkets and a cookery book, *Mea-*

sure for Measure by Elizabeth Reilly, has been written for "families with a diabetic in them".

The connection between over-consumption and obesity or diabetes is easy to appreciate. That between over-consumption and coronary disease is more obscure. In fact, nobody knows for sure how sugar consumption leads to coronary disease (if it does). But statistics seem to point that way, since increased sugar consumption (eight times higher now than 150 years ago) goes hand in hand with increased coronary disease, and the appearance of such disease at an earlier age.

The correlation applies not only to the white races who constitute the wealthier societies of the world, but to Indians, Africans and American negroes who have adopted a sophisticated diet in recent years. The authors compare sugar consumption of Indians in India with Indians in Natal, rural Zulus with urban Zulus, Yemenis in Yemen with Yemenis in Israel, and show that freedom from saccharine disease is not a racial characteristic but a state that exists in people whose consumption of refined carbohydrates is low. When the same people increase their consumption, their susceptibility to coronary disease, diabetes and other "civilised" ailments increases also. Sugar is the villain of the piece in most cases, but refined starch in the form of white rice affects the incidence of diabetes in India.

However, we need more than correlations to make much headway with a theory, and the next step is to attempt to show that alteration in diet can cure or arrest a diseased condition. The most striking example related by one of the authors was that of a man of thirty-six who had a heart attack while playing hockey. His blood cholesterol was found to be twice the accepted safety limit. Refined carbohydrates were cut but no restriction was placed on fats. In eight weeks the cholesterol was down by half, and remained down despite a fairly high intake of saturated fats.

Though the authors do not consider animal fats in a natural state have any bearing on coronary disease, they suggest that what they call unnatural fats may have. By this they mean fat in a form not found in nature but disguised in a readymade food such as chocolate, cake or ice cream, where fat is associated with sugar.

2. *Removal of fibre*

As well as causing unnatural concentration of carbohydrates by decreasing the bulk, removal of fibre also leads to tooth decay. Refined flour becomes sticky when moist, clinging to the teeth and changing, through fermentation, to acid which attacks the enamel. With sugar the process is even more rapid. Historically it can be shown that tooth decay has gradually increased over the years with the refining of flour, which started to some extent in very early times, but has dramatically increased with the more recent refining of sugar. Tooth decay is not generally regarded as a disease, or even as a possible cause of digestive trouble, but is accepted philosophically as a fact of life, like a November fog.

The second result of lack of fibre in the diet is colonic stasis, which means a slow progress of food residue through the large intestine. Though there may not be noticeable constipation, the effect over the years may be varicose veins and/or diverticular disease. Of the first, one may ask, ''what's the connection?'' and the second, ''what is it?''

Naturopaths have long held that varicose veins are caused less by standing, tight garters or weak blood vessels than by pressure on the iliac veins adjoining the large intestine caused by accumulation of slow-moving food residues. These large veins receive blood from the leg veins and any pressure on them causes a back pressure which strains the valves of the leg veins. Weak valves, therefore, are not the prime cause of varicose veins but a step along the way. The cause is a faulty diet. The authors of *The Saccharine Disease* uphold this view.

Diverticular disease is one of those things which have sneaked up on us quietly. Without any publicity or dramatic manifestations, it can nevertheless cause quite a lot of trouble in later life. It is said to afflict a third of all people over sixty.

What is it? A diverticulum is the medical name for a sac or bulge formed in the wall of the intestine by the pressure of excess food residue forcing the lining through the muscular wall. In time the sacs may become focal points for bacterial infection leading to peritonitis. Deaths from this cause have increased more than ten times during the last fifty years.

3. *Removal of protein*

Carbohydrate foods—wheat, rice, potatoes, sugar beet—all contain a proportion of protein, usually around 10 per cent. This amount is reduced during refining and in the case of sugar, removed altogether. The authors suggest that a small amount of protein is necessary at all times to buffer the gastric juice and protect the mucous lining of the stomach. Without it, gastric juice can attack the lining and cause ulcers.

Medical opinion has always considered excess gastric acid to be the main cause of ulcers, but the authors, continuing their evolutionary standpoint, deny that evolution could have allowed such a situation. The trouble (which is of recent origin anyway) is much more likely to be caused by some outside agency such as the consumption of unnatural foods. The fact that other proteins may be taken at the same meal as refined carbohydrates does not help because, according to the authors, food is not evenly mixed but remains in layers in the stomach; therefore any refined component, particularly a helping of pure sugar, stimulates acid production without providing the necessary buffering action.

The claim is supported by some interesting geographical instances. For example, the "ulcer belt" in India follows the consumption of factory milled rice; Japan, where both white rice and sugar are eaten, has the highest ulcer rate in the world; during World War II, ulcer rates in Japanese prison camps varied according to the supply of milled rice; on the Russian front, the incidence of ulcers in the German army declined as the troops moved east towards Stalingrad, away from sources of refined foods.

Throughout the book, the authors are at pains to prove, from statistics, that diseases of civilisation are practically non-existent in countries where people still eat unrefined foods, and that during the two world wars deaths from these diseases dropped in other countries also. This, they claim, was due to food rationing, which gave us a smaller amount of sugar.

As in the case of diabetes, it is logical to assume that all the saccharine diseases take some time to develop, and the authors give a round figure of twenty years as the average. Thus, most of these diseases will show up in middle age or later. Tooth decay is an exception.

So we can see that the usual fatalistic pessimism which regards illness in later life as inevitable, is nonsense. You are not ill because you have reached forty or sixty, but because you have been mismanaging your diet for a certain time. As the authors state, in their final word of advice: "People are prepared to take endless trouble over the maintenance of a motorcar, but over the maintenance of that infinitely more delicate mechanism, the human body, they are seldom prepared to take any trouble at all."

The second book about diseases of civilisation—*Pure, White and Deadly* by John Yudkin—deals entirely with the dangers of refined sugar, and in particular with the argument that sugar, not saturated fat, is the main contributor to coronary thrombosis.

Professor Yudkin also supports the idea of an evolutionary basis for diet; but he believes that early man was a carnivore and therefore that a diet high in animal fat is natural. So he rejects the theory that animal fats can be responsible for coronary disease. Since it seems likely that early man obtained his carbohydrates (which made up a small part of the diet) from fruits rather than roots, he probably preferred sugar to starch, and the present-day sweet tooth is something inherited from the distant past.

With the introduction of agriculture about ten thousand years ago, cereals and palatable starches were more easily obtained and the carbohydrate portion of the diet increased. This change in diet is described as the first of two food revolutions. The second food revolution, which is comparatively recent, concerns the artificial juggling with food made possible by technological ·advance. These artificial aspects include refining, the use of chemical fertilisers, factory farming and the manufacture of convenience foods.

In the author's opinion flour refining does not matter at all. In this he disagrees with the authors of *The Saccharine Disease* and many others. Chemicals and factory farming are similarly blameless; in this he disagrees with many ecologists. But the refining of sugar is another matter. Sugar consumption has increased eight times during the last 150 years, and while total carbohydrate remains steady, the sugar proportion has shot up while bread consumption has fallen.

Because palatability and nutritional value no longer go together as they did in primitive times—flavours can be manufactured—what we want is no longer the same as what we need. What most people want is sugar, sugar and more sugar, and because refined sugar is an artificial substance, this can be disastrous.

The arguments, as in the first book, are supported by correlations between sugar consumption and disease in various countries and by experiments. The South African evidence (Indians in Natal and Zulus) is quoted, also that of the Yemeni immigrants into Israel, who show an increase in disease after twenty years of sugar eating, though their fat consumption remains the same as before. Two other examples are given—the people of St Helena, who eat only moderate amounts of fat but a lot of sugar, have a high incidence of coronary disease; the Masai and Samburu tribes of East Africa live on milk and meat, so their fat intake is high, but they eat no sugar and have no coronary disease.

Since national averages can be misleading, investigations were made with individual patients and it was found, by questioning, that patients in the hospital with heart trouble had a history of higher sugar consumption than those hospitalized for other reasons.

The next step was to see whether increasing the sugar intake of animals or human volunteers produced any of the symptoms normally associated with coronary disease. These include high blood cholesterol, high level of triglycerides (natural fats), high level of insulin and increased stickiness of blood platelets. In the case of animals, all these were found, plus atheroma of the main artery as well in cockerels. In the case of healthy human volunteers, the changes were induced temporarily in some cases, disappearing soon after the diet reverted to normal. But in most cases the only consistent change was in triglyceride level—the other changes were not found. This leads to the conclusion that not all people are equally susceptible. Women, who get less coronary disease, are not susceptible until after the menopause, which implies that hormones come into the picture. Professor Yudkin is, in fact, convinced that sugar leads to coronary disease by upsetting the hormone balance of the blood in some way not yet understood.

Other diseases mentioned as having a correlation with sugar intake are obesity, diabetes, indigestion, dental decay, imperfect sight, skin trouble, gout and possibly cancer. Of these, indigestion is of most interest to the man in the street since it is already the subject of much do-it-yourself treatment by patent medicines. The answer, apparently, is simply to cut down on sugar. The effect was discovered accidentally in the case of overweight patients who noticed an improvement in digestion as soon as they started to diet. Professor Yudkin himself says that after suffering from indigestion most of his life, he became accidentally cured while dieting to lose weight. After this, tests were made on a number of patients and the results confirmed in 70 per cent of the cases.

The theory is quite simple. Sugar irritates the digestive tract on account of its high osmotic pressure. As we may remember from school biology, a solution with a high osmotic pressure draws water from one with a lower osmotic pressure when the two are separated by a membrane such as a cell wall. The osmotic pressure depends on the number of molecules in the solution so substances with small molecules (and therefore more of them to a given volume) have a high osmotic pressure.

Sugar is one of these, and in drawing water from the cells of the stomach lining it sets up an irritation. Starch, having large molecules, does not have this effect. So we see that this theory conflicts with the ulcer theory advanced in *The Saccharine Disease,* which implicates refined starch also, and for a different reason.

Pure, White and Deadly concludes with a strong appeal for the banning of all sugar, brown as well as white. Brown sugar is 99 per cent refined, only the final stage being omitted. So people who think brown sugar is ''raw'' and therefore a natural food are deluding themselves. The only slight advantage brown sugar (and honey) may have is that it contains trace elements such as chromium and you cannot easily eat so much.

These two books, which agree in many of their conclusions but disagree quite a lot in the theories leading up to them, represent the case against sugar as a factor in coronary disease. But the fat theory retains a larger following amongst scientists as well as among the public who have heard of cholesterol but have not heard the sugar story at all. How firm the scientists are in their stand can be shown by the fact that 7 April 1972 was World Health Day—The Day of the Heart. The April issue of the UNESCO *Courier* was devoted entirely to articles by medical experts from all over the world on various aspects of heart disease. And not one single mention was made of sugar.

The fat theory of coronary heart disease has been around for many years. The ''coronary'' or heart attack is a result of a clot in a coronary artery, which supplies blood to the heart muscle. If the artery is narrowed by fatty deposits (atheroma) the clot can cause a complete blockage, cutting off the blood supply and causing the death of part of the heart muscle. This does not necessarily mean the death of the patient. He can recover and carry on with a partly damaged heart muscle, though a scar remains. The danger lies in a recurrence, for it is probable that all the coronary arteries are equally affected and further clots (breaking off from the fatty deposits) are likely to form.

It is generally agreed that these fatty deposits consist mainly

of cholesterol which has somehow "gone wrong". Cholesterol is a fatty substance absolutely essential to life, being a
constituent of cell membranes and nerve sheaths. In addition
to what is taken in the diet, the liver manufactures it. So
cholesterol itself is not undesirable, only its presence as a
deposit on the artery walls is. If it has been deposited as a result
of excess amounts in the bloodstream, how has this excess got
there?

It is generally thought by proponents of the fat theory, that
blood cholesterol levels depend on the proportion of total
energy derived from fats. The affluent countries are character-
ised by a high intake of calories (overeating) of which a high
proportion (40-50 per cent) is fat; of this, the main part is
saturated fat and cholesterol. It is in affluent countries that
coronary disease is rampant, and a morbid fear of cholesterol
has led to such kinky activities as eating poached eggs without
the yolks.

Supporters of the fat theory admit that there is a correlation
between sugar intake and heart disease but suggest that since
fats and sugar are often eaten together in the form of cakes,
biscuits and ice cream, the correlation is unimportant. How do
they account for the good health of fat-eating pastoral tribes in
Africa, and the Eskimos? They don't. The Masai, they say,
have become adapted to a high cholesterol diet, which unkind
critics might say was begging the question. The Eskimos are
not referred to at all.

A strong point in favour of the fat theory is the fact that
manipulation of the diet can alter blood cholesterol concentration; saturated fats raise it, polyunsaturates decrease it. This
has led to a mad rush for the salad oil bottle and a switch to soft
margarines in place of butter.

A number of secondary factors also come into the picture.
These include smoking, stress, high blood pressure and lack of
exercise. But the doctor's vague murmurings, "cut smoking,
calm down, take a holiday, get some fresh air and exercise",
fall on deaf ears. Human nature likes its cures quick, easy,
preferably out of a bottle and certainly without exercise.

Supporters of the fat theory and the sugar theory are at loggerheads. Since the fat theory has by far the greater following, its supporters give only a superior smile when sugar is mentioned. The sugar people, representing a voice crying in the wilderness, are more sensitive, and a whole chapter of Professor Yudkin's book is devoted to the infamies of those who won't listen to him.

So with this battle raging, it is interesting to come across a couple of theories which reconcile the two opposing sides. First, we have Dr Michael Crawford's theory of the importance of structural fats, which is much more than a mere offshoot of the fat story. His book, with its rather unmemorable title *What We Eat Today,* stresses the importance of essential fatty acids and suggests that modern eating habits have led to a deficiency of EFA in the diet—they have been cut by half during this century.

This idea itself is not new—it was put forward by Professor H. M. Sinclair (the leading authority on EFA) nearly twenty years ago. Sinclair was the first to suggest that EFA in combination with cholesterol forms cell membranes and nerve sheaths; without sufficient EFA, cholesterol is useless and so accumulates on the artery walls. Dr Crawford takes the argument a step further, claiming that surplus cholesterol is only deposited on the artery walls if the walls themselves are first weakened by EFA deficiency. Artery damage is the cause, not the result, of atherosclerosis.

The two simple essential fatty acids, linoleic (found mainly in seeds) and linolenic (found mainly in leaves) are built up by animals into more complex long-chain forms. The carnivore gets these complex forms "ready-made" and so is able to develop a better brain and nervous system.

How has modern eating led to a shortage of structural fats? The author makes these points:

1. With increased population, man came to depend more on concentrated foods and less on fruits and vegetables. The affluent societies took to eating more protein and fat,

primitive societies depended on high carbohydrate cereals or bananas. Both lead to imbalance.

·2. As crops are forced, for high yield and rapid growth, they contain less EFA. (The oil content of wheat is much less than it used to be.) The same applies to livestock; fast growth means less time to construct the long-chain fatty acids. Meat from factory farm animals consists of more fat than protein but only a fiftieth of the fat is unsaturated. The meat of a wild animal consists of more protein than fat and a third of its fat is unsaturated.

3. Refining of cereals removes the oil. Breakfast cereals have no oil content compared with old fashioned porridge. Cakes, biscuits, and ice cream are often made with saturated fat. Saturated fat is not in itself objectionable (it is a source of energy) but its increased consumption today means that the structural fats have been pushed out and the balance upset.

It is this imbalance which is thought to cause the trouble. Whereas the fat theory and the sugar theory are both concerned with high blood cholesterol as the cause of atheroma, Crawford suggests that a breakdown of the artery wall, due to lack of EFA, comes first. Fibrous patches with calcified plaques appear, then clots and fatty deposits build up on these, first as "fatty streaks" then as atheroma. But without the original artery weakness, atherosclerosis would not occur. Since both excess saturated fat and excess sugar lead to EFA deficiency and artery breakdown, the two opposing theories can be reconciled. They are both right, though possibly not for the reasons their supporters would advance.

Practical proof comes from a surprising quarter—wild animals in Africa. With the restriction on their habitat caused by an expanding human population and overcrowding in game parks, elephants have been forced to take to a diet largely of grass instead of trees. This has apparently reduced the EFA in their diet and autopsies show arterial disease together with ·symptoms of premature senility. Since elephants are not concerned with smoking, keeping up with the Jonses or lack of exercise, these findings point to a change of diet as the major cause of arterial disease.

A further point made in Dr Crawford's book is the importance of a balance between the two basic EFAs which he calls the seed kind (linoleic) and the leaf kind (linolenic). Since it is easier to get the first in the form of corn oil, sunflower seed oil and soft margarine, those people who have become interested in EFA are likely to be getting it in an unbalanced form. (Monkeys fed an unbalanced mixture show disease, which clears up when the balance is restored.) Dark green leaves, usually discarded from salad, are the best source of linolenic acid.

A second theory which reconciles the fat and sugar schools comes from Dr H. G. Bieler, whose philosophy is outlined in Chapter VII. He blames not one or the other, but the combination of the two cooked together which, he thinks, produces an ''impure cholesterol''

We have been told that cholesterol is essential for the manufacture of cell membranes among other things. Dr Bieler thinks it forms part of the smooth artery lining itself. A fast flowing stream erodes its banks, but the bloodstream does not erode the artery walls as long as they have a strong, smooth lining, made from pure cholesterol, which is constantly renewed. But when the lining is made from ''impure'' cholesterol it wears out faster than it can be renewed, lumps break off and form clots and the lining becomes roughened.

Eat any kind of fat you like, says Dr Bieler, only eat it in its natural form. Don't cook it up with starch or sugar and eat it as potato chips, cake, biscuits or ice cream.

Circumstantial evidence supports the theory. Heavy fat eaters, such as the Masai and Eskimos, remain healthy. Affluent societies, who eat both fat and sugar cooked together, are the ones with heart disease.

White bread, smoking, and chlorinated water are responsible for heart disease according to Dr George Stanton, author of *Health Hazards of a Western Diet*. If this book is dismissed as extreme, it will be less on account of its theories than its style, for it is a diatribe. Dr Stanton is anti nearly everybody, from scientists and fellow medicos to naturopaths; from big business to pseudo-health food pedlars and those who believe them. This attitude unfortunately sets up a certain sales resistance in the reader, so that the facts which are being hammered into our heads tend to melt away in their own heat.

In general, the book supports *Saccharine Disease* theories. It is only the heart disease theory which is new. Based on work done by Dr J. A. Price, this theory claims that it is only in the presence of chlorine that fatty deposits are laid down on the artery walls. Otherwise, a high fat diet and high blood cholesterol would not lead to artery damage. Since chlorination of water has existed for about one hundred years and chlorine dioxide has been added to white bread for about twenty years, the corresponding increases in heart disease during these periods is accounted for.

Dr Price conceived the idea after noting that milking apparatus cleaned with a chlorine germicide acquired a "milk-stone" deposit. He then experimented with chickens, giving them a fatty mash with chlorinated water, and found deposits in their arteries after a few weeks. The controls, given distilled water, remained healthy.

The chlorine in the water is inactivated by boiling or by calcium. This accounts for the lower incidence of heart disease in hard water areas and also (according to Stanton) accounts for the apparent immunity of women—they drink their water boiled, with tea or coffee.

Returning to the starch side of the picture, we find that the work of Cleave, Campbell and Painter has been followed up by an investigator who considers lack of fibre the most important factor in diseases of civilisation. D. P. Burkitt (a surgeon working for the Medical Research Council) in a paper entitled "Some Diseases Characteristic of Modern Western Civilisation" points out that carbohydrate refining has affected diet in two ways—excess starch and sugar consumption on the one hand and reduced fibre intake on the other. While the authors of *The Saccharine Disease* stress the first aspect, Burkitt stresses the second.

It seems that we now only eat half as much bread as we did one hundred years ago and this half contains only a fifth the amount of bran it used to. Packaged cereals have replaced porridge. So altogether we eat less than a tenth the fibre the Victorians had. The result of all this is colonic stasis with its end-products diverticular disease, appendicitis, bowel cancer, varicose veins, ulcerative colitis and hiatus hernia. In this, the author is simply supporting the arguments set out in *The Saccharine Disease.* But turning to coronary heart disease and gall bladder disease, he continues to blame fibre depletion.

The theory is that bile acids and cholesterol are re-absorbed by the colon when fibre is lacking in the faeces. It has been suggested by other research that this leads to raised blood cholesterol. Cholesterol stones associated with gall bladder disease may be similarly involved. Here we have yet another example of similar conclusions being reached by a different route.

Mental troubles, we are told, are on the increase, and you don't have to be a statistician to see that violence certainly is. Can diet possibly have anything to do with it? J. I. Rodale in his book *Natural Health, Sugar and the Criminal Mind* says yes. His collection of case histories indicates sugar as the cause of most of our sociological ills. If some of the ideas sound a bit way out (Ivan the Terrible and Hitler were both sugar addicts) we have to admit that the arguments are based on the same methods as the books by scientists we have just been discussing, i.e. a correlation between sugar intake and anti-social behaviour, plus experimental evidence that when sugar is cut out of the diet of individuals (usually obstreperous children) their behaviour reverts to normal. This is scientific reasoning, and if we accept it from the experts we must accept it from the amateur too.

Rodale points to the increase in juvenile delinquency, student unrest, vandalism and senseless criminal activities and equates these with the rise in sugar consumption by young people, who live on soft drinks, ice cream and drug store snacks. He suggests that delinquency is often associated with broken homes, not because the home is broken but because the children of such homes tend to congregate in drugstores. Sugar gives them energy—even its opponents agree on that—and energy without a positive outlet leads to violence. And we have to remember that McCarrison's rats, fed on the British working man's diet (which included jam and sweet tea) became cannibals—just about as anti-social as you can get!

On the experimental side, the book cites several cases of children whose personality problems have been cured by changes in diet. He suggests that criminals usually have a record of high sugar consumption. He asks for more investigation into this, but as one might expect, the authorities find the idea too cranky.

To sum up, we may say that these authors, most of them medically qualified, are convinced that many of our civilised ailments are due to refined or unbalanced foods. And if none of them has so much as mentioned vitamins or minerals as being missing, we can find plenty of reformers who think these deficiencies may be the most important of all.

D I A L O G U E

Q. *What is the connection between stress and heart disease?*
A. Originally, stress meant danger. The primitive response to danger was fight or flight. On receiving a stress signal from the adrenals, the body prepares to protect itself by, among other things, pouring sugar and fat into the bloodstream as a source of energy, constricting the blood vessels so as to speed circulation, and increasing the supply of cholesterol, possibly in readiness for repairs to injury (cholesterol being a constituent of cell membranes). If violent action took place, all these factors were utilised and once the emergency was over, body chemistry returned to normal. But if no violent action takes place, tension is not released and body chemistry remains permanently in a state of alert. High blood pressure and

cholesterol persist and in fact increase with every new stress. The state of emergency can be cancelled most easily by physical action, which is what it was designed for. But failing this, the official advice on protection against heart disease can help to some extent as follows:

1. Cutting consumption of saturated fats and/or refined carbohydrates helps most, since these substances in the bloodstream stimulate the production of cholesterol by the liver. (Cholesterol in the diet is not thought to have so much bearing on the matter.)

2. Cutting smoking helps by allowing blood vessels to relax. Smoking is not only an artery constrictor but a stimulant in itself, having much the same chemical effect as a primitive danger warning.

3. Consumption of PUFA helps reduce existing blood cholesterol by combining with it for building purposes.

4. Increasing fibre in the diet speeds up the passage of residue through the intestine and so lessens the likelihood of cholesterol in the faeces being re-absorbed. Also, the fibre itself absorbs cholesterol and so aids its excretion.

5. It has been noted that coronary heart disease is less widespread in hard water areas, but just how hard water helps is not known. According to Dr Stanton the answer would be: calcium inactivates chlorine which he believes is one of the main causes of atheroma.

6. Reduction of uric acid helps since urates build up on the fatty deposits in the artery walls. (See under arthritis, Chapter VI dialogue.)

7. It is also suggested that lecithin, described as an emulsifier and transporter of fat, helps by breaking down large globules of cholesterol and "moving it on", so that deposits are less likely to accumulate. Lecithin is a phospholipid, differing from a triglyceride in that one of its three fatty acids has been replaced by phosphoric acid. It occurs in food, and though lost in refining can be made by the liver, provided the ingredients (EFA, choline and inositol) are

present together with vitamin E for protection for vitamin B6 and magnesium which are part of the enzyme needed for synthesis. The action of lecithin is speeded up by methionine, an amino acid. So people who stress the teamwork aspect of diet point out the EFA alone is not the answer—you need seven items to keep excess cholesterol from piling up. Quite apart from the difficulty of remembering the seven items and where they come from, it seems more logical to avoid having excess cholesterol in the first place.

8. Some research suggests that vitamin C lowers cholesterol levels. Since vitamin C is to some extent an antioxidant like vitamin E, it could act in the same way, by protecting EFA and so putting cholesterol to constructive work.

The answer seems to be the ultra simple one of balancing exercise with food intake, with the accent on unrefined, unconcentrated foods which retain their EFA, and the avoidance of too frequent stimulation by smoking, alcohol and coffee. The avoidance of stress, always so glibly recommended, is impossible, but the release of the tensions caused by stress is easily accomplished through exercise. Regular exercise throughout life seems to give complete protection— the Masai and other pastoral tribes with a high fat intake have no heart trouble. Even as a cure exercise can help. A few enlightened doctors are now introducing their heart patients to a system of exercise, very gradually and under strict supervision.

Q. *Since many cholesterol-containing foods also contain lecithin, why the worry?*
A. Eggs, which contain a lot of cholesterol, also contain lecithin, but not enough to balance. But many people think that it is not so much diet cholesterol we should avoid as saturated fats which stimulate the production of cholesterol by the liver.

Q. *If we eat cholesterol, why would the liver continue to make it?*

A. Possibly because the process is automatic, particularly in response to a stimulus. However, it is thought that over a long period, the amount in the diet does affect the amount synthesised, which is why the Masai, who live on a high fat diet, produce very little. But this is a long-term adaptation—you cannot switch off the synthetic process by suddenly altering the diet. This idea of adaptation is behind the breast feeding theory. Since breast milk has a high cholesterol content, production by the liver is not unduly stimulated and remains low throughout life. Bottle-fed babies need to produce their own cholesterol at a higher rate and continue to do so throughout life.

Q. *Is the taking of extra PUFA, the most widely adopted remedy, effective?*

A. A belated "cure" can never be as effective as prevention, but for those who suddenly find they can't walk up hill, this remedy seems to work. Though EFA in the diet is essential for healthy arteries according to Dr Crawford, this is quite different from taking large dollops of PUFA after the trouble has developed. Here, nutritionists issue a warning. Too much PUFA may be worse than too little, according to some research, causing premature ageing. This theory is based on the fact that in moderate quantities, natural oils have sufficient vitamin E to protect them (safflower oil is an exception) but with larger quantities (something to do with surface area) the amount is not adequate, and extra must be taken. If this is not done, then the PUFAs may be oxidised and will end up doing more harm than good, forming by-products which cause cell breakdown. How do you know what is enough? Since there is no agreement on the basic requirements of vitamin E, you don't. Adelle Davis suggests taking an extra 100 mg of vitamin E with every tablespoon of oil. Other estimates suggest a 50 per cent increase with a "high PUFA intake" (what is high?) but on a very much lower basic dose. We have to accept the fact that the requirement is simply not known, estimates varying from under 20 mg a day on the part of orthodox science, to several hundred from those enthusiasts who consider vitamin E "the greatest discovery in one hundred years".

Q. *What is the difference between arteriosclerosis and atherosclerosis?*
A. Arteriosclerosis was the term originally used to describe hardening of the arteries, at one time thought to be the principal artery disease. It is caused by loss of elasticity plus mineral deposits in the middle layer of the artery wall, resulting in high blood pressure. If a hardened artery ruptures (usually a capillary in the brain) a stroke results. About a quarter of all deaths of cardiovascular origin are from strokes. Atherosclerosis refers to the fatty deposits, mainly consisting of cholesterol, on the inner surface of the artery wall, restricting the size of the tube. A clot breaking off from the deposit may block the artery. Atheroma may also become hardened by minerals. Both conditions, by restricting the size of the arteries, contribute to high blood pressure, a disease now so common that it is taken for granted in middle age. The Australian Heart Foundation estimates that 10 per cent of the total population of Australia has high blood pressure. But in primitive people, the blood pressure does not increase with age. Food reformers think this points to diet as a cause.

Q. *Has coronary heart disease really increased so much recently, or has it simply had more publicity?*
A. The increase is very real and very alarming. In America it is said that CHD kills 1,300 people a day—more than all other illnesses combined. In Britain, there are now six times as many deaths from CHD annually as there were before World War II. The links with diet are: fat consumption has increased from 33 per cent to nearly 50 per cent of the diet in Britain since 1948. It is now above the danger level. Due to intensive farming the ratio of saturated to unsaturated fat in meat is

increasing without the consumer realising it. (Faster growth means less time in which to build up complex PUFAs.) Sugar consumption has almost doubled this century and the sale of ice cream (which combines fat and sugar) has increased fifty times in the last fifty years.

At the same time, exercise has declined with increased affluence. Children who once used to walk or ride bikes to school are collected by bus; they watch TV when once they would have played out of doors. Of a recent batch of army recruits found unfit for basic training, 60 per cent were overweight.

As we have seen from the geography of CHD, it is a disease of affluent societies. It seems likely that the three factors—changes in diet, reduction in exercise and the rat race—all combine to bring it about.

CHAPTER VI

MORE ABOUT DEFICIENCIES

THE LAST CHAPTER has shown that it is not only cranks ·and faddists who are worried about modern trends in diet, but respected scientists and research workers as well. Though individual theories may differ, with one voice they condemn refining.

We saw that there have been two major periods of change in the history of food for the human race—first, the coming of agriculture about ten thousand years ago, and secondly the entry of technology into the world of food a mere one hundred years ago and increasing every day. The first made more food available and the second makes what there is stay available longer—by juggling around with food we can prevent it going bad and so cut down waste; we also cut down the time people have to spend preparing meals.

But, say food reformers, you can't get something for nothing; in gaining convenience, something is thrown away. That something is the living part of our food, which is essential for health, and the items most often lost are vitamins and minerals.

There has probably never been a time when we could talk happily about vitamins. When there were plenty of them, we didn't know about them; now we know about them they seem to be disappearing. What is the cause of this lack? The answer, say food reformers, is the technology of convenience—longer shelf life which makes things easier for the merchant, and packaged, prepared dishes which make things easier for the housewife.

What exactly is a vitamin? More books have been written about the subject and more mental indigestion caused than by all other aspects of nutrition put together. So many facts are presented that by the time you get to the bottom of the page you've forgotten what was at the top. There are long lists of the sources of each vitamin, long lists of what each one does inside you and still longer lists of what will happen if you go short of any of them. Many of the symptoms are common to all—fatigue and dizziness for example (only equalled by the fatigue and dizziness you get from reading about them). So it is not surprising that you get glassy-eyed long before the end of the book and your mind is a blank as soon as the last page has been turned. Works from authoritative sources are quite simply text books, and even those with a lighter touch still read like an auctioneer's catalogue with a few jokes put in to keep the audience awake. Small wonder that most of us know as much about vitamins as about the political situation in Nicaragua.

However, if we want to keep the family healthy, we need to know the story in broad outline, without going into too much detail. A vitamin, we are told, is something that in very small quantities is essential to life. This rather vague and unsatisfactory definition (which could apply to trace minerals also) is the best the experts can do, because the different vitamins have very little in common, either chemically or in function. Unlike minerals, they have complex molecules and unlike enzymes they cannot be manufactured in the body and have to be taken in food. The exceptions, as we have seen, are vitamin D, which can be made by the action of sunlight on the oils of the skin (though it occurs in food also), and some of the B vitamins which are synthesised by bacteria found in the intestine.

Just to recap what we said about vitamins in Chapter II, some, or maybe all, vitamins go in families or complexes and new members are still being discovered. The B group consists of at least twelve members, the E group of eight and the K group of perhaps ten. The B and C vitamins are water soluble;

they cannot be stored and need to be taken every day. The rest, being fat soluble, can be stored for a few weeks.

Vitamins do a whole lot of different, unrelated jobs. Some of the B vitamins are involved in the metabolism of carbohydrate, vitamin C with the formation of connective tissue (the material between the cells) and the neutralisation of poisons, vitamin D with the absorption of calcium and phosphorus, vitamin E with the integrity of essential fatty acids and vitamin K with blood clotting.

It is indicative of orthodox medicine's concern with disease rather than health that the names of vitamins as taught to school children refer to the diseases they prevent rather than their positive functions. Thus vitamin B1 (thiamine) is termed the anti-beri-beri vitamin (on TV it is the happiness vitamin!); niacin (another of the B complex) is the anti-pellagra vitamin; vitamin C is the anti-scurvy vitamin and D is the anti-rickets vitamin. Yet how many of us have the faintest idea what beri-beri, pellagra and scurvy are?

Beri-beri is a disease of the east, found amongst very poor people who eat white rice and not much else (rice polishing, in fact, led to the discovery of thiamine, in the Dutch East Indies); pellagra occurs amongst corn eaters in the southern USA.

The story of scurvy is fairly well known. We learn that it is what sailors get if they don't take plenty of lemons on board with them. The British were the first to discover the value of lemons or limes and British sailors used to be known as limeys. Some unkind people say this is what made the British navy great—not the ships, not the guns, not the admirals, but the fact that there were always plenty of sailors around to fire the guns. It was not until the lemon ration had been in effect for a hundred years or so that vitamin C—ascorbic acid—was actually synthesised (1932).

With rickets we come nearer home. Vitamin D being required for the metabolism of calcium and phosphorus to make strong bones, a lack in childhood causes softness and consequent deformity of the bones. This has been taken care of in recent years by adding vitamin D to baby foods. However, rickets may still be found in poor communities where vitamin D in the diet is inadequate *and* there is a lack of sunlight to help its formation in the skin. This is why rickets used to be associated with city slums.

Vitamin D occurs in fish liver oils, butter and margarine, but otherwise is not richly supplied in food. The amount needed by adults is comparatively small and the fact that it can be made by the action of sunlight on the skin keeps the average person just about topped up. But the elderly, who do not go out of doors, are often deficient. A mild deficiency leads to malabsorption of calcium resulting in brittle bones. Rickets, banished in this country for many years, is now thought to be creeping back. Could TV addiction, keeping children indoors even on sunny days, have anything to do with it?

Vitamin A, being unconnected with any dramatic ailment, is sometimes called rather vaguely the anti-infection vitamin, because it is concerned with the health of skin and mucous membrances, where infections may develop. But doctors dismiss the idea that the vitamin can stave off infection. Experiments with rats suggest that trebling the normal dose (no danger of poisoning) increases the lifespan. Rather better known is the fact that vitamin A affects the speed of the eye's adaptation to poor light.

Vitamin A is only found in animal foods, the richest source being fish liver oils, though some occurs in milk and butter. But vegans need not go short, for it can be manufactured by the body from carotene, found in green and yellow vegetables. In green vegetables, the yellow colour is masked by chlorophyll.

Mention a more recent discovery, vitamin E, and the first reaction is usually a giggle, for the tie-up with sex and fertility was its first claim to fame and the label has stuck. However, there's much more to it than that. It is now known that in addition to being an important component of the endocrine glands (pituitary and adrenals as well as the sex glands) vitamin E is an anti-oxidant and so protects the unsaturated fatty acids from oxidation, enabling them to play their part in building arteries, nerves and cell membranes. (See Chapters II and V.) This anti-oxidant property has given vitamin E the description "oxygen sparing". In other words, the less oxygen wasted in combining with fatty acids, the more there is available for other purposes. This is especially important to heart cases whose blood supply (and therefore oxygen supply to the cells) is impeded by narrowing of the arteries.

Most of the work implicating vitamin E in the relief of heart trouble has been done over the last thirty years at the Shute Institute in Canada. Although all the staff are specialists (Dr Evan Shute is an outstanding surgeon and gynaecologist) they are often called quacks by those who find it hard to accept their results.

There was a time when the word "deficiency" automatically meant vitamin deficiency, but it is now realised that minerals may be lacking in refined foods. This aspect received less publicity at first (except for iron pills which have been with us for decades) but, staunchly supported by manufacturers of supplements, it is now catching up.

We have to bear in mind that there are two main groups of minerals:

1. Those which constitute part of the body structure and so are needed in measurable amounts, for example calcium and phosphorus in bones and teeth, sodium and potassium in body fluids, iron in the red cells of the blood, etc.
2. Those which act with enzymes, or are involved in hormone production, or whose function is not really understood. These are the trace minerals, and though the amounts needed are tiny, they are essential (Chapter II). But they are toxic in excess.

Those minerals which form alkaline salts are sodium, potassium, calcium and magnesium. Minerals which form acids are phosphorus, sulphur and chlorine. Since the blood is normally very slightly alkaline, excess acids are neutralised by alkaline salts which act as buffers. Alkaline minerals constitute what is known as the alkaline reserve, and since we tend to eat a preponderance of acid-forming foods, many food reformers think these are the minerals we need most.

Since the whole subject of deficiencies is controversial, it is a complex subject, and its very complexity plays into the hands of big business. For the housewife, if she is at all interested in nutrition, is faced with three choices:

1. She can buy books, study the subject and use her judgement.
2. She can buy supplements and trust that the manufacturer has got the answer right.
3. She can decide that nature knows best, which means buying whole, compost-grown foods.

The first solution is the one the commercial types know we are too lazy to adopt.

The second solution demands a blind faith in science, a susceptibility to advertising and a belief in the magic of pharmaceutical products. Most people have all these requirements and this is the most popular line of action amongst those who think about health at all.

The third solution is the one behind food reform, but even here there are pitfalls. People who never heard a cock crow or saw the early morning dew on the cabbage patch are only too eager to tell us all about natural goodness—at a price. In Chapter VIII we will try to find out how near "health foods" can get to satisfying the back-to-nature concept. But first let us look more closely at the practices which are said to be threatening the value of our food. These are:

Reduction in soil fertility (dealt with in Chapter IV).
Refining and processing (partly dealt with in Chapter V).
Long distance marketing.
Wasteful cooking methods.
Consumption of destructive substances.

Refining

Refining is done for two reasons—to make a more attractive-looking product (white bread, white sugar, white rice) and to extend the shelf life of the product.

The aspect of refining which causes most heated argument (on the part of both attackers and defenders) is that of flour. The wheat grain, as we know, consists of the germ, which will grow into a new plant, and the endosperm or starch upon which the germ lives until it has produced its own roots and leaves. The whole thing is contained in a husk.

Flour made from the whole grain is brownish in colour and, since it is a live food, is liable to be attacked by insects; the germ oil is somewhat unstable and sooner or later will go rancid in contact with air. It is therefore a better commercial proposition to remove the germ and bran and feed them to animals. Most people prefer white bread anyway. In so doing we lose most of the vitamins (mainly B and E), the minerals and oil, and not least the fibre. (See Chapter V.)

In enriched white flour (which is what we have had ever since World War II), two of the B vitamins are put back, together with iron and calcium. At this news, food reformers give a hollow laugh, for twenty things, they say, have been taken out of flour and only four put back, in an unsatisfactory form.

The chemists' answer to this complaint is that all the remaining missing nutrients are freely available in other foods, so not to worry. But as more and more foods become refined, this sounds to the critics like starry-eyed optimism. Until recently it was assumed that minerals at least could be made up from vegetable sources. But the claim (not proved to the satisfaction of scientists) that chemical fertilisers adversely affect the make-up of crops (Chapter IV) means that an increasing number of agitated town dwellers are heading for the health food stores to buy compost-grown vegetables or bottles of pills.

The vitamin B part of the story is the subject of two points hotly debated. Bread is a mainly carbohydrate food (though it contains 10-12 per cent protein) and carbohydrates need some of the B vitamins for their metabolism. If you eat a carbohydrate such as sugar, which contains no vitamin B at all, the body will do its utmost to get hold of the vitamin from somewhere. Since B is water soluble it is not stored for any length of time, so extra supplies must be taken from some temporary source, with resulting shortage for other purposes. So every time you eat white sugar or white rice you are digging into your small reserves. Some of the carbohydrate you eat will have to remain only partly processed. One of the half-way products of carbohydrate metabolism is pyruvic acid. Normally this is broken down to provide energy, but if it has to stay around in acid form it irritates the nerves and may affect the heart muscle. It also interferes with the absorption of calcium. So people deficient in vitmain B are, according to food reformers, nervous, irritable and lacking in energy.

This theory is dismissed by orthodox scientists. Pyruvic acid, they agree, does irritate the nerves and cause fatigue—in fact this is an early symptom of beri-beri. But if sub-clinical symptoms such as irritability and lack of energy were due to B deficiency, there would also be cases of beri-beri in the community as well. You are unlikely to get the half-way stage without at least some cases of the complete disease. No, there is plenty of vitamin B around—in enriched white bread, meat, and all over the place.

The second talking point about vitamin B is that it is a complex of maybe twelve to fifteen members. The best known are thiamine (B1), riboflavin (B2) and niacin. These are the ones usually in synthetic vitamin B pills, and they are also added to enriched white flour. But what about the rest? Do they matter? The powers that be obviously don't think so, but food reformers think that the complex must be treated as a whole and balanced as in the natural state (whatever that may be). The taking of some B complex members without the others may actually cause a deficiency of the missing members after a time, just as pulling the choke of your car, which alters the proportion of gasoline to air, can only be a temporary measure. Orthodox scientists dismiss this theory also. The members of the B complex are not chemically related, they say. They are only grouped together by accident because all are water soluble co-enzymes and they usually occur together.

Those who feel deprived by the loss of vitamin E and its accompanying oil from white bread can, of course, buy wheat germ or eat breads made from white flour with added germ. Since nobody knows how much vitamin E we need, orthodox scientists are on safe ground in saying there's plenty around in other places (some of them even deny it's necessary at all). If we accept the "official" estimate of five to twenty international units a day, there probably is. But if we accept Dr Shute's estimate of several hundred units a day, there obviously isn't. It all depends on who you believe.

Those who are convinced of the importance of fibre (Chapter V) can, believe it or not, buy bran by the bag. Or they can eat bran bread made from stone-ground wholewheat flour. Since these loaves contain no additives, they lack the spongy texture of white bread and go stale sooner. But the nutty taste is said to make up for this drawback, according to the one per cent of the population who eat them.

Another aspect of refining is that of vegetable oils. Since the importance of polyunsaturates became known (Chapter V) there has been a brisk trade in salad oils other than olive oil which is only mono-unsaturated. These include sunflower seed, sesame seed, safflower seed and corn oil. Linseed oil is so unstable that it is not a commercial proposition as a food, but is used as a quick-drying agent in paint.

Oil can be extracted from the seed either by cold pressing or by using a chemical solvent with heat. This method enables more oil to be extracted, but some food reformers say it destroys vitamin E and the more unstable of the fatty acids— only cold pressed oils are any good. But go to a health food store and try to get cold pressed oils and you draw a blank.

Manufacturers of chemically extracted oils (who supply health food stores as well as supermarkets) say everything is quite all right, nothing has been lost. Safflower seed oil, however, contains insufficient vitamin E to protect it so a synthetic anti-oxidant has to be added. Synthetic anti-oxidants do not find favour with food reformers.

The final aspect of refining which worries many critics is the pasteurisation of milk. Although the process is necessary as a safety measure to get rid of bacteria when milk from many sources is pooled, it destroys some vitamins, minerals and enzymes and, according to reformers, results in an altogether inferior product. Riboflavin (B2) is not affected by heat but is destroyed by light when the glass bottle stands on the door-step. Since milk is a major source of B2, this is quite a point. But those who advocate dark bottles are regarded as cranks.

Pasteurised milk contains no vitamin E. Even raw cow's milk contains only a fraction of that of breast milk, so bottle-fed babies get off to a bad start. Some think this bad start affects the individual's susceptibility to heart disease in later life. The La Leche League aims to publicise this theory and get mothers back to breast-feeding their babies. Perhaps in blaming vitamin E deficiency they are missing the point. It is the structural fats in breast milk (protected by vitamin E) which go to make strong arteries.

Is raw milk safe? Only if it is certified. If you live in the country and know the right farm, you may be able to get it. Town dwellers haven't a hope.

Long distance marketing and preservation

If there's many a slip twixt cup and lip there are even more twixt farm and lip in these days of Hungarian plums and Chinese rabbits. Somebody has worked out that the average supermarket cabbage you buy in a supermarket is six days old. To a nation long since resigned to eating eggs three weeks old, six days may seem positively juvenile. But we are told that the vitamin C content lasts only three days. Under optimum growth conditions, i.e. heat and moisture, the enzyme which builds up vitamin C during the growth of the plant, starts to destroy it once the plant has been harvested. Contact with air, bruising and wilting also cause loss of vitamins. Fruits and vegetables with thick skins do not suffer in the same way as leafy greens, but the practice of picking fruit unripe to compensate for travelling time means that nutrients are still below optimum level when the fruit is sold.

These varying conditions all make nonsense of the food tables you find in books on nutrition, telling you how many milligrams of this and that there are in a slice, helping or cup of a certain food. Even supposing you had the patience to work out the number of slices or spoons needed to give the recommended daily allowance, the answer could be 100 per cent off owing to conditions of transport and storage you know nothing about.

With trade agreements stretching ever wider and produce coming from ever more distant places, the snags involved in long distance transport of perishable goods are bound to increase, even with refrigeration. What we stand to lose most is the easily destroyed vitamin C.

Vitamin C is probably the best known of the vitamins. Most people, however vague about the rest, know that C occurs in fruit and vegetables, which is why greens are ''good for you'' and that if you don't get enough you will get more colds and possibly other infections. Oddly enough vitamin C is only a dietary requirement in primates and guinea pigs; other animals make their own.

It is now known that vitamin C plays a part in the formation of collagen, the cement or connective tissue which binds cells together. When it goes missing you start to fall apart, as in scurvy, or to a lesser extent in pyorrhoea. It is also said to combine with the toxins produced by bacteria and viruses, neutralising them, which is where the cold cure side of its reputation comes in. However, despite the findings of several research workers which indicate that vitamin C in large doses can replace antibiotics in the treatment of infections, medical opinion remains sceptical.

Recent research suggests that vitamin C reduces the level of cholesterol in the blood.

Those who believe in vitamin C's antibiotic powers, led by Nobel Prize winner, Professor Linus Pauling, point to the fact that primitive man must have had far larger quantities in his diet than we do today. From this it is concluded that the tissues should be permanently saturated and we should think in terms of grams, not milligrams, of daily dose. Though the USA has for some time fixed its MDR (minimum daily requirement) at 75 milligrams in contrast to the 30 mg in Britain, Dr Pauling's ideas are not accepted by medical opinion as a whole. Now it seems the US is about to abandon the saturation idea and reduce its recommended dose. Russia, however, sticks to 200 mg a day.

When time and distance involved in marketing have stretched to breaking point, we fall back on preservation. The main methods are:

Heating
Drying
Chemical preservatives
Canning
Quick freezing
Freeze drying

1. Heating kills bacteria direct, as in pasteurisation or sterilisation.
2. Drying by sun, smoke or hot air kills bacteria by dehydrating them. Spray drying in a vacuum preserves vitamins, otherwise some of the B and C vitamins are lost.
3. Chemical preservatives include the old-fashioned ones, salt and sugar, which kill bacteria by osmosis. The strong solution draws water from the weak, so killing by dehydration, even in a liquid. Acid is also a preservative— hence pickling. The most common of the modern preservatives are sulphur dioxide and benzoic acid. Although objected to on principle by health food addicts, both occur in nature. Sulphur-dioxide destroys vitamin B1, so may not be used in any food which is an important source.
4. Canning involves the heating of vegetables in a salt solution and fruit in a sugar solution, usually a syrup. After

removal of air the can is sealed, heating continues for maybe half an hour more, then it is cooled rapidly, forming a partial vacuum so that oxygen content is low. The losses are mainly of vitamins C and B1, which are susceptible to heat, and minerals. Some of the vitamins and minerals remain in the liquid. After cooking, canned vegetables retain about a third of their vitamin C.

5. Quick freezing has now replaced ordinary freezing, since by this method the cells are not destroyed by the ice crystals. On thawing, the product regains its original form. However, it must be used quickly; 90 per cent of the vitamin C disappears an hour after thawing. The nutrient losses are somewhat less than in canning.

6. Freeze-drying involves the drying at very low pressure of a quick-frozen food. The ice sublimates to vapour without a liquid stage, so no refrigeration is needed and the product regains its original form and flavour as soon as water is added. The method is expensive—four or five times that of freezing or canning—and is used mainly for expeditions.

All these methods involve a compromise between the ideal of eating fresh food and the practical necessity of keeping a largely urban population supplied with a wide variety of food all the year round. Those who yearn for the "healthy" past forget that a few decades ago very little variety was available during the winter months and the only year round source of vitamin C in reasonable quantity was potatoes. Until the eighteenth century not even potatoes were available.

Wasteful cooking methods
If refining, transporting and storage are robbing us on the one hand, perhaps we are saving some nutrients by more enlightened treatment in the home. A generation ago, greens were boiled to a pulp more often than not and vegetables were left to wilt because we didn't have refrigerators. Now, most people beware of over-cooking, the continental influence has

made us more salad conscious, and almost everyone has a refrigerator. The vitamin content of frozen foods is said to be higher than that of "fresh" (several days old) produce in the grocer's, though not as high as that of something from your own garden.

Even with fresh foods, we can still waste a lot of goodness by careless treatment such as prolonged washing, excess peeling, exposure of cut surfaces to air, bringing greens to the boil from cold instead of plunging them into boiling water, adding soda, prolonged cooking, cooking without a lid and keeping food warmed up. The exposure to air part also applies to freshly made juices and to canned citrus juices (the best of the canned products as far as keeping vitamin C goes). Both must be used right away or they lose much of their goodness. It isn't often that laziness is an advantage, but if you are too lazy to peel potatoes (as I am) you retain the precious vitamin C which is most concentrated just inside the skin.

Cooking mistakes are nothing new; we cannot blame them on technology, and it seems probable that they are on their way out at least as far as the housewife is concerned. But large-scale catering is another matter. Cooked food served in restaurants, cafeterias, schools and even hospitals is bound to be more or less worthless as a source of vital nutrients.

Consumption of destructive substances

The last hazard is the newest and the least thought about. Food reformers say we lose most of our vitamins, sometimes all, by combining them with destructive substances such as:

Mineral oil laxatives which remove the fat-soluble vitamins A, D, E, and K.

The well-known preservative, sulphur dioxide, destroys vitamin B1. It is not allowed by law in foods which are a major source of B1, but is found in most packaged and canned goods, beer, cider and sausages.

Alcohol destroys B and C.

Antibiotics and sulfa drugs, by destroying the bacteria which synthesise vitamin B in the intestine, temporarily deplete supplies. Hence the depression which often follows an illness. Yet few doctors prescribe extra B along with antibiotics.

Sleeping pills (barbiturates and narcotics) destroy B. This makes the person taking them even more jittery, so more pills are needed.

Coffee and tea (caffeine), which are diuretics, cause B to be excreted. By stimulating the production of adrenalin (which all stimulants do) they also use up C.

Aspirin is said to destroy C.

Smoking is said to destroy C to the tune of about 25 mg (one orange) per cigarette, so a smoker needs several times his official daily dose. This theory is not officially accepted.

Worry, by increasing brain activity, uses up sugar and therefore B, and by increasing the flow of adrenalin, uses up C. The same applies to other stresses such as anger, anxiety and frustration.

Chlorine dioxide, the preservative in white bread, destroys E.

Iron destroys E, which should be taken several hours before or after an iron supplement.

Rancid fats destroy E.

Chlorinated water destroys E.

Light destroys B2, therefore milk in glass bottles standing in the sun has lost most of its supply. Milk is the main source of B2.

Of the fourteen items on this list, most of us take eight or nine fairly frequently and probably at least six every day. Yet we are assured that deficiency is unlikely in affluent countries.

Here are some possible causes of mineral deficiency (for further explanation, see dialogue).

Mineral	*Cause of deficiency*
Potassium	Lack of fruit and vegetables in diet Consumption of excess sodium, mainly table salt Consumption of refined sugar Caffeine Lack of magnesium Cooking in water Worry Diuretics
Iron	Caffeine Oxalic acid
Magnesium	Alcohol Chemical fertilisers in soil
Calcium	Caffeine Too much or too little protein Excess sodium; Oxalic acid (in spinach and rhubarb) Excess refined carbohydrate Pasteurised milk Lack of vitamin D Excess fluoride
Trace minerals	Refining Chemical fertilisers in soil

So much for deficiencies. Now what about poisons?

D I A L O G U E

Q. *Is the view that we get adequate vitamins in food widely accepted?*
A. Yes, certainly for the average adult. It is agreed that pregnant women, nursing mothers, children and the elderly may not always get enough, but the rest of us are said to get ample supplies in ordinary, everyday foods. One text book for students states that only six of the approximate total of over thirty known vitamins are of interest in nutrition (meaning possibly connected with disease). The requirements of B6 are not known so it is rarely referred to. At the other end of the scale we find claims that the average American is slightly deficient in twenty or more nutrients, just getting along without being vitally healthy. Since most town dwellers feel in a run-down condition, it is not surprising that this doctrine has tremendous appeal. Is there any scientific proof? Dr Geoffrey Taylor, whose speciality is vitamin deficiencies, claims that 25 per cent of his elderly hospital patients are short of vitamin B and 90 per cent are short of vitamin C. But elderly hospital patients are not average.

A few years ago, a local Health Department worked out an average diet and added up the vitamins A, D, B1, B2, niacin and C (but not E). In all cases the diet supplied considerably more than the recommended minimum. No convenience foods were included. Many alternatives were given, so that a person who opted for fruit instead of sponge cake, or salad instead of macaroni, would come out with a different total. But since the meals were of the hearty home-cooked type, there would be little likelihood of a deficiency of any nutrient, provided the vegetables were not over-cooked.

Q. *What is meant by the statement that vitamins must be taken in the correct balance?*
A. This is usually said about the B complex, because the B vitamins, being co-enzymes, are concerned with metabolism,

so it is thought that stepping up one without the others might upset the balance. (This does not tie up with the statement that excess water-soluble vitamins are automatically eliminated.) The argument is most often put forward by food reformers, but the orthodox *Manual of Nutrition* also states, regarding vitamins in general (not only the B complex), "Balance is essential. If one deficiency is treated, symptoms of the others may appear."

Opponents of the view point out that vitamins occur in haphazard proportions in different foods. Since we do not know what the ideal proportions are (requirements in many cases are not known), and even if we did, we would not know how to supply them, there is not much to be done about it. Instinct may have taken care of the situation once, but it does so no longer.

At this point the commercial people jump on the bandwagon, with a multi-vitamin/mineral pill to take care of all the calculations for us—perfect health in a handy, convenient minipackage. This might be all right if, *(a)* we were all the same, and *(b)* there was any agreement on the recommended doses. But we are not all the same. Our eating habits differ, so our deficiencies (if any) differ also. This problem is one more argument in favour of a balanced diet of wholefoods, which would automatically include the right proportions of vitamins and minerals without any calculations being needed.

Q. *Has the interaction of vitamins with each other been proved?*
A. It has not been proved that treating one deficiency will cause others to develop. But it is generally accepted that vitamins work together synergistically, i.e. each one increases the efficiency of the others. Experiments with rats have shown that 80 per cent of those supplied with the whole B complex were resistant to disease, whereas only 20 per cent of those given the incomplete complex survived. In the human field, more rapid recovery from pellagra was noted with the whole B

complex than with niacin (the anti-pellagra vitamin) alone. Similarly vitamins A and D support each other, and in most deficiency conditions several nutrients are needed for best results.

Q. *What is the argument for natural versus synthetic vitamins?*
A. Chemically, they are identical since the chemical formula is the same in both cases. Those who are against synthetic vitamins suggest that in nature there is also some minute quantity of an extra ingredient, too small to be identified, which may act as an inhibiting factor, controlling the rate of release. The synthetic version, with no control, is too potent and therefore less effective. Some manufacturers of synthetic vitamins agree with this theory and are producing "gradual release" versions.

Q. *Can the existence of this "extra something" be proved?*
A. Some research involves the process of chromatography. The fact that dyes absorb chemicals at different rates means that substances can be analysed by means of coloured patterns. The patterns made by some natural and synthetic vitamins are different, indicating that the chemical make-up is different although the known parts may be identical.

Q. *What vitamins are dangerous in excess?*
A. As far as we know, only A and D. This was discovered when both were added to baby formulas. Warnings were issued and steps were taken to ensure that formulas which might overlap did not contain potentially dangerous quantities. Needless to say, the doses for babies are much smaller than for adults. The quantities which would be poisonous in adults are at least forty times the normal for vitamin A and ten

times the normal for vitamin D, so overdoses are unlikely in adults taking supplements according to the instructions on the bottle. Cranks may kill themselves, as shown by a case in 1974 of a man who took vast quantities of vitamin A tablets daily in addition to quarts of carrot juice.

Q. *Why are the lesser members of the B complex left out of most supplements and generally regarded as unimportant?*
A. Vitamin B12 is acknowledged as very important by all schools of thought. Without it, you get pernicious anaemia. Since the requirement is very small, most people have no problem. But since B12 only occurs naturally in animal foods, vegans may go short unless they avail themselves of special supplies produced from bacterial cultures. But since the importance of a vitamin is judged by what happens if you don't have it, those not associated with spectacular ailments tend to be dismissed. Some are concerned with grey hair, and who cares about that? A slightly more controversial member, pyridoxine or B6, known to be required for the metabolism of proteins and fats, is now sometimes included in supplements. It is lost during flour refining but can be obtained from various foods including meat, eggs and health foods such as yeast and wheat germ. The daily requirement is not established so nobody is unduly worried about a shortage except those who suspect that as part of the team which utilises cholesterol, it may be more important than we think.

Pantothenic acid, known as the anti-stress vitamin (a wonderful selling title if the stuff was on sale) is rarely included in supplements, probably because it is very widely distributed in protein foods. The remaining members of the complex are in a constant state of flux, for some which were included have now been promoted to a status of their own with new letters, and new members keep turning up. However, as long as you like liver there is no problem, for there is not a single known B vitamin that is not found in it.

Q. *Why are the B vitamins more publicised than any other?*
A. Probably because their beneficial effect is most striking—
you become "a new person" within a few days of treatment.
This is no doubt due to the mental and psychological effect;
the B complex is associated with nerve health, mental health,
confidence and courage, a description to make any hardheaded scientist wince, but supported by innumerable examples.

As we know, thiamine (B1) is concerned with carbohydrate
metabolism and the release of energy, so it is logically enough
"the pep vitamin". A deficiency means that sugar is not
properly utilised so the subject develops a craving for sugar
which only makes matters worse. Sugar is the food of the
brain, so improper sugar metabolism affects brain, nerves and
personality. Since worry increases brain activity, vitamin B is
further depleted. Niacin is described as "the courage vitamin". Deficiency is said to cause "suspicion, hostility,
apprehension and depression". Biotin restores optimism and
improves mental well-being according to American research
workers. Small wonder that the depressed and nervous victim
of the rat race seeks solace in the "happiness" pill.

Q. *If B vitamins are added to bread, do we not get enough*
without supplements?
A. The amount in bread is more than enough to deal with the
starch in bread, but whether you have enough altogether
depends on other factors such as how much sugar you eat, how
much you fret and fume, whether you take sleeping pills etc.
Refined sugar is the main depleter of vitamin B, so if you eat
more than other foods can provide for, then there is a deficiency. The problem has increased despite fortification of
flour, say food reformers, on account of vast sugar consumption, the frequent use of antibiotics for minor ailments and the
extensive use of sleeping pills. Vitamin B is fairly widespread
in small amounts in protein foods, but apart from liver, the
richest sources (yeast and wheat germ) are not foods in the

normal sense. No one eats yeast for pleasure (though maybe we shall have to one day, when we have run out of space for growing crops) and wheat germ appeals mainly to faddists; it is unlikely to challenge snap crackle pop as a breakfast food.

Q. *If white bread is fortified, in what way is wholewheat bread thought to be superior?*
A. The bread argument is not new—it has been around for well over a hundred years. Food reformers claim that far more has been taken out of bread than is put back; twenty nutrients, they say, have been removed as against four added. The losses include the lesser B vitamins, vitamin E, minerals, lecithin and EFA. As well as retaining most of these things, wholewheat bread has protein of slightly higher biological value.

Those interested in learning more can read the early story in *Breads White and Brown* by R. A. McCance and E. M. Widdowson. Though written about twenty years ago, this book is still the bread "bible", found on the bookshelf of everyone in the industry. We learn that two of the earliest crusaders for wholewheat bread were Sylvester Graham early in the last century and Dr T. R. Allinson towards the end of the century. Graham was an American clergyman and vegetarian with a large following, who campaigned for natural foods. His bread was eaten for years by health addicts. It was known that the discarded part of the wheat grain contained protein, fat and minerals (vitamins were not yet on the map) but there were two objections to its inclusion:

1. The faster passage of wholewheat through the digestive tract, owing to the laxative action of fibre, meant less time for absorption of nutrients.

2. The proportion of phosphorus to calcium was thought to be unfavourable to bone development.

The stalemate lasted until Dr Allinson gave wholewheat a further boost during the last years of the century. He was an unorthodox doctor, a vegetarian teetotaller who was struck off the register for campaigning against drugs. He continued to run a Nature Cure practice and being dissatisfied with the quality of bread available, started to mill his own flour. His company is still flourishing today.

Meanwhile roller milling had made white flour even whiter, which suited everybody—the public who liked it that way, the farmers who needed the germ and bran for their livestock, and the millers who made more money by selling to both parties.

During World War I, bread in Britain became slightly browner, to spin out wheat supplies. In Denmark, drastic measures were taken. Hindhede, the Minister of Food, decided to slaughter all the pigs and some of the cattle to conserve wheat stocks for the population. He attributed the fall in death rate from disease during the war to this measure.

After the war, bread became white again but by now vitamins had appeared on the scene and there was much interest in the importance of vitamin B. McCarrison's lectures led to a movement of both scientists and cranks in favour of wholewheat bread.

During the 1930s there was growing official interest in the matter. The League of Nations recommended an increased extraction rate—more germ and bran in flour. Just before World War II fortification was discussed at an international conference but action was postponed by the war.

Just after the war Professor McCance and Dr Widdowson decided to settle the argument of brown versus white by practical experiment. They chose groups of children from German orphanages and fed them with (1) wholewheat bread, (2) fortified white bread, and (3) unfortified white bread, all with added chalk. Bread made up the bulk of the diet, the rest consisting mainly of vegetables and soup. Vitamins A, D and C were given. To everyone's surprise, the children grew equally fast in all groups, which gave the answer "white bread is just as good as brown".

Perhaps it might be more accurate to say "white bread is just as good as brown as a growth promoter". Growing children need protein above all; there is practically no difference between white and brown bread in protein content; as there was plenty in the diet, all children got sufficient protein for growth. The missing nutrients in the unfortified white bread might have been made up from the vegetables. So we are still back to square one regarding the merits of white and brown bread over the years, particularly for those who do not eat many vegetables.

One of the snags of brown bread was long thought to be the presence of phytin in the bran, which as phytic acid could combine with calcium and iron, rendering them unavailable. Later findings showed that the body could adapt to the presence of phytin and restore calcium balance. Possibly this adaptation may take some time, for troubles with immigrants, who eat wholewheat *chappattis,* are now being reported. This could be due to their relatively lower reserves of vitamin D due to less sunshine in their new surroundings.

It may come as a surprise to learn that three of the four items added to fortified white flour are not considered essential after all:

1. Vitamin B1 is the most important ingredient lost during refining, so fortification is necessary.

2. Niacin can be made from the amino acid tryptophan. Apart from this there is more than enough in a normal diet. Those vitamins complained about but not restored (B6, pantothenic acid, biotin, vitamin E) are readily available in other foods.

3. Calcium was added because it was thought the extra phytate in bran would limit the absorption of calcium. It is now known that man can adapt, so the addition was never really necessary. Chalk is now added to white bread for quite a different reason—to protect the heart (see hard

water, Chapter V). But perhaps it makes more sense to add calcium to water rather than to bread.

4. Iron is added, not to offset milling losses, but as a mass medication to counteract the many cases of sub-clinical anaemia. However, the type added is not well absorbed. Excess iron causes liver damage, so mass medication is not a good idea—iron should be given according to individual needs.

Q. *What is the mystique about stone-ground flour?*
A. The heat generated in stone grinding distributes the germ oil and flavouring evenly throughout the flour, so that even if the bran is sieved out later, all the germ oil will remain. With roller milling the germ is squashed flat instead of being finely ground, so is easily removed by sieving. This means that stoneground flour of 81 per cent extraction would contain more germ oil than roller milled flour of the same extraction. It also contains slightly more bran.

Q. *What is the evidence concerning vitamin C and colds?*
A. The evidence is divided between those who swear by it (from practical experiment) and those who scorn the idea as ridiculous. An article in the British Nutrition Foundation Bulletin (September 1973) states: "The tendency to ascribe to vitamin C functions other than the simple prevention of scurvy has produced a rich harvest in terms of unsubstantiated claims and untested hypotheses." The writer waxes indignant at the vitamin's association with cholesterol, bone formation, arthritis and cold prevention. But why should a vitamin have only one function? Let's look at the cold cure story first.

It is based on the theory that vitamin C is a de-toxifier, combining with toxic substances so that both are excreted, and in large doses acting as an anti-biotic. If this is correct, then it would of course clear up any infection.

The man behind the cold prevention theory is Linus Pauling, biochemist and Nobel Prize winner. Both he and his opponents admit that there is a mass of conflicting reports. But whereas Pauling sums up the findings in favour of his theory, others give the verdict "no satisfactory evidence". However, several hardheaded anti-crank doctors and nutrtionists treat their own colds with vitamin C, some on a "no harm in trying" basis, others completely convinced.

Since the battle is likely to rage for some time, the only way for the individual to settle it is by personal trial. The main thing, as with any trial, is to be thorough, otherwise the trouble may be "too little, too late". Most people wait until they are sure they have a cold before taking anything. The time to act, we are told, is when the first tickle is felt in nose or throat. Then you take 600 mg and repeat every three hours until cured. Since most people forget the three-hourly dose, it is not surprising that positive proof is hard to come by. And how do you judge results? Can you say, "My cold would have been worse without vitamin C", or, "My cold would have lasted longer without vitamin C"? Comparisons are not really possible, but if you find that time and again a cold fails to develop, at least it looks hopeful.

Q. *What about the other alleged properties of vitamin C?*
A. The anti-oxidant action of vitamin C on cholesterol was mentioned in Chapter V. The evidence comes from several separate studies in Canada, the USA and Czechoslovakia.

The connection with bone formation comes from the widely accepted view that vitamin C assists in the formation of collagen, or connective tissue strength. (With a breakdown of connective tissue, we get scurvy.) Collagen is said to bind calcium and phosphorus in the bones; when it becomes too weak to hold the minerals, bones lose their strength.

The arthritis theory really concerns rheumatism, since arthritis involves mineral deficiency also. If the collagen of the capillaries breaks down, haemorrhage results and cells which normally would have been supplied by those capillaries die and become a focus for infection. If this happens in a joint, inflammation will result. It is also suggested that if the connective tissue in general is weak, bacteria from other points of infection may migrate through it to the affected spot to aggravate the condition, hence the theory that bad teeth aggravate rheumatism. Records indicate that rheumatic fever has been cured by massive doses of vitamin C. But those who become too enthusiastic about the vitamin C megadose idea are warned that excess could lead to the formation of oxalate stones.

Q. *What is vitamin P?*
A. This is the bioflavanoids which occur with vitamin C and are thought to affect the permeability of the capillaries. The two vitamins are thought to act synergistically, backing each other up so that each increases the efficiency of the other. Vitamin P is not included in synthetic vitamin C tablets.

Q. *How much of the vitamin E story is officially accepted?*
A. Practically nothing beyond its connection with fertility in animals. Even its function as an anti-oxidant, protecting EFA, is still queried by some scientists. However, the importance of vitamin E in vegetable oils is recognised (to prevent rancidity, not to aid health). Despite the Shutes' work over the last thirty years, positive experimental proof of man's need for vitamin E is said to be lacking. A doctor writes: "No one has shown that a lack causes any diseases in man or that giving extra vitamin E has any beneficial effect at all." There is a strong view that proof concerning animals does not constitute proof concerning people. This is because animals often have different enzymes and physiological processes. To be accepted, experiments on humans have to be controlled. This means that controls, who do not get the treatment, must exist alongside those who do. It is not so easy, with serious illness such as heart trouble, to

deliberately withhold treatment from half the patients, just to prove a point.

Vitamin E, dubbed "the rejuvenation vitamin" by enthusiasts, is said to do these things:

1. By protecting EFA it strengthens blood vessels (which need EFA in their structure) and by preserving EFA to combine with cholesterol, it prevents cholesterol deposits.

2. By protecting EFA it prevents the formation of destructive substances resulting from oxidation of EFA, which cause cell breakdown and premature ageing. Vitamin E has been shown to increase the lifespan of rats.

3. Because of the anti-oxidant function, there is an oxygen-sparing effect—the amount breathed in goes further. In theory this should be useful to athletes, mountaineers at high altitudes and people with partially blocked blood vessels.

4. Needed by the endocrine glands, it aids hormone production.

5. Helps destroy poisons from pesticides, additives and drugs by inducing detoxifying enzymes in the liver.

Points 1 and 3 explain the benefits claimed in heart cases. Point 2 explains the anti-ageing theory, though the human case is unproved. Premature ageing is much too vague to be established. Point 1 also explains the claim that vitamin E improves varicose veins. Point 4 explains the link with fertility, and since the pancreas is also an endocrine gland, reports that vitamin E cures or alleviates diabetes fit in here. Point 3 supports a claim that Olympic teams given extra vitamin E did better than comparable teams without it. But how do you decide on comparable teams? This test is disputed by other investigators. A Scottish football team was given vitamin E by a diet-conscious coach. This is described as "modern black magic" in *Human Nutrition and Dietetics* by Davidson and Passmore.

Those who wish to run up mountains, fix their varicose veins or live to a hundred, are advised to curb their enthusiasm and build up the dose gradually. Doses of over 200 mg a day taken suddenly may cause a rise in blood pressure which could be dangerous to those whose blood pressure is already on the high side.

This is still the most controversial vitamin. There is hardly a thing you could say about it which would not be violently contradicted by someone.

Q. *What has happened to vitamin F?*
A. It has disappeared. This was the old name for the essential fatty acids, which were termed a vitamin because it was thought that only very small quantities were needed—approximately 1 per cent of total fat intake. Now the amount thought desirable is much larger—some say a third of total fat intake.

How many essential fatty acids are there? If you read three different articles on the subject, you probably get three different answers, because the experts don't seem to agree. Originally there were three—linoleic, linolenic and arachidonic. Later one or other of the last two, or both, were knocked out on the grounds that the body could build them up from linoleic. Dr Crawford (see Chapter V) thinks we need the first two in equal quantities, but nobody else seems worried. Linoleic acid comes from seed oils and is found in soft margarine and salad oils.

Q. *What minerals are most likely to be deficient in food?*
A. Minerals are widely distributed in food, but can be lost in cooking, canning or refining. It is said that 95 per cent of the alkaline minerals (which we are liable to need most, on a predominantly acid diet) may be lost in cooking water, depending, of course, on how you cook. Save the cooking water to add to soup can help. It is suggested that cooking

losses may even turn otherwise alkaline vegetables into acid foods.

Iron is the mineral most commonly deficient anywhere in the world. The reason is not so much shortage in soil or food, as difficulty of absorption. On an average only half of what is present is absorbed; in some foods the amount may be as little as 10 per cent. It is thought that a large number of women are actually deficient or on the borderline. The association between iron and haemoglobin and hence energy, leads a number of people to think that if they feel tired they must be anaemic. Energetic advertising on the part of the iron pill industry encourages the idea. Yet anaemia may have other causes, and do-it-yourslef therapy is not advised. (It is thought that excess iron can cause liver disease.)

Adelle Davis has an uncomfortable theory that shortage of vitamin E leads to breakdown of red blood cells. Since iron destroys vitamin E, any treatment of this type of anaemia with iron would only make things worse. Since individuals vary so much, suspected deficiency should be checked by an expert and treated accordingly.

Calcium is perhaps the most controversial mineral. There are three views: (1) that deficiency is unlikely except among children, pregnant women, nursing mothers and the elderly; (2) that calcium deficiency is more widespread than that of any other mineral, and (3) that calcium can do harm. This last view, which is a minority one, is based on the fact that calcium deposits are found on the artery walls in cases of artery disease. Calcium, we may remember, goes 99 per cent to bones and teeth and 1 per cent to the nerves. The main source is milk and milk products. The deficiency theory is based on factors which inhibit calcium absorption:

1. Lack of vitamin D, magnesium and B6 which make up the rest of the absorption team.
2. Destruction by pasteurisation of the enzyme phosphotase, causing calcium to be precipitated. This is dismissed as nonsense by scientists but supporters of the

theory claim that calcium is precipitated in pasteurisation tanks, and that calcium is precipitated in pasteurisation tanks, and how else did it get there if not from the milk?

3. Excess phosphorus, found in high protein foods including those taken for their vitamin B content such as liver, yeast and wheat germ. The excess phosphorus, having nothing useful to do, has to be excreted as calcium phosphate, depleting the calcium reserves. (If this was the case, it would prove the impossibility of trying to manipulate the diet artificially. You take vitamin B for your nerves, get too much phosphorus, lose calcium and so end up as before!) Recent research indicates that adequate protein aids calcium absorption, but too much or too little causes excretion.

4. Excess carbohydrate, by stimulating the alkaline digestive juices, hinders calcium absorption, which needs an acid medium. Pyruvic acid, the half-way stage of carbohydrate metabolism, however, renders calcium insoluble.

5. Excess use of alkaline salts (anti-acids or laxatives), has a similar result, by neutralising stomach acid. Also chlorides and fluorides, including table salt.

6. Oxalic acid from spinach and rhubarb renders calcium insoluble.

7. Phytic acid, present in whole grains, was at one time thought to combine with calcium and iron, making them unavailable. This was for a long time a big argument against wholewheat bread, although some phytin is broken down by yeast during baking. Now, however, it is thought that we all possess a phytin-splitting enzyme, enabling us to adapt to high phytin. Phytic acid was thought to cause rickets in Dublin children suddenly given wholewheat bread during the war. The alarming increase in rickets led to a panic return to white bread, but the limiting factor may have been vitamin D. People living on wholewheat in the tropics, where there is plenty of sunshine, do not seem to suffer from calcium defi-

ciency, but immigrants from the tropics to Britain do, suggesting that the adaptation may take time.

The reasons why calcium so often "goes wrong" are still a mystery. Why do we get deposits in arteries, joints, muscles and tissues, making for stiffness and old age diseases? If this is not due to excess calcium, what is the cause? Adelle Davis suggests that when cells break down, calcium is deposited in the tissues. Lack of vitamin E may cause cell break-down by allowing EFA in cell walls to be oxidised. So vitamin E deficiency is at the back of the calcium deposit problem. It's a theory on its own, with no support, but nobody seems to have a better one.

Two other minerals which food reformers feel concerned about are potassium and magnesium. Magnesium is part of the calcium team, and with B6 is part of the enzyme which synthesises lecithin. Although it is only needed in small quantities, its absence from the teams can interfere with metabolism. In theory there should be no shortage, for magnesium is part of the chlorophyll molecule and therefore present in all greens. But it can be lost in cooking water and excreted in alcohol.

Potassium is the mineral most likely to be deficient in those who hate fruit, vegetables and salads and like a lot of salt. It is said to be needed for muscle contraction and for producing energy from glycogen in the muscles. Potassium and sodium exist in solution in the body fluids, sodium mainly outside the cells and potassium within the cells. The two have to be in balance; excess sodium upsets the balance; in sea salt, the sodium is balanced to some extent by other minerals. Herbivores need to balance their high potassium intake by taking extra sodium—hence the need for a salt lick. As with other minerals, the main causes of deficiency are lack of fruit and vegetables in the diet, and bad cooking.

Q. *What is the connection between minerals and arthritis?*
A. Despite frequent statements that arthritis is incurable, some

types at least have been completely cured by mineral therapy under the Nature Cure system. Latest research on arthritis suggest that there are three types:

1. Osteo-arthritis, which is mechanical in origin, caused either by injury or faulty posture. Joint cartilage is damaged and extra bone is produced to take its place, roughening and distorting the joint. Potassium is thought to play some part, not understood, in controlling the formation of extra bone.

2. Rheumatoid arthritis, which is chemical in origin. The trouble is thought to be malfunction of the adrenals which are unable to supply cortisone. The result is inflammation of the joint capsule. Injection of synthetic cortisone brings only temporary relief with many side effects. The aim is to get the adrenals back to normal, and this, it is claimed, can be done by means of minerals, mainly potassium. Some trace minerals are needed too but it is not known which are the most important. Herbalists all have their theories, and to be on the safe side seaweed products, which contain all minerals, are often prescribed.

3. Gouty arthritis is caused by excess uric acid which combines with sodium to produce chalk-like deposits of sodium-biurate which cause grating of the joint and may also affect the arteries in conjunction with cholesterol. This condition can also be helped by potassium and other minerals.

Many cases of arthritis consist of combinations of the above types. Because of the danger of artery deposits in the last type, patients are advised to take steps to reduce cholesterol, which includes cutting animal fats.

Q. *Which trace elements are important for diet in general?*
A. Very little is known about trace elements or what they do.

The amounts needed are extremely small and they are toxic in large doses. Copper, for instance, destroys vitamin C on contact. It is claimed that chemical fertilisers hinder the absorption of trace minerals by the plant. The importance of traces in the soil is shown by the story of cobalt. A mysterious livestock disease was noticed in some areas of Australia and New Zealand. Sheep and cattle began to fade away for no reason that anybody could discover. After years of worry and frustration it was found that the soil lacked even the smallest trace of cobalt, the mineral associated with vitamin B12. Only a few ounces per acre were needed to make the land support healthy livestock again.

CHAPTER VII

MORE ABOUT POISONS

W E S A W I N Chapter I that the poison story has mushroomed somewhat since the days of the old auto-intoxication idea. Now the worriers tell us that poisons are coming at us from three directions; from the farm (in the form of pesticide residues), the factory (in the form of additives), and from inside our own bodies (due to mistakes in eating).

The pesticide story centres round DDT and the chlorinated hydrocarbons which are to some extent recognised as dangerous. It all started with *Silent Spring* by Rachel Carson, a book in the bombshell class which produced violent reactions, both for and against. The battle continues to rage, the chemists' argument being that we need that extra 10 per cent of the world's crops which insects allocate to themselves. But science can't win, for as fast as new pesticides are developed, insects manage to become immune to them. This gives an opening to food reformers to press their point, suggesting that we might as well call a truce with the pests for the sake of good health.

How is health affected? Is DDT a poison? It certainly is to a creature the size of an insect, but doctors say there has never yet been a case of human illness attributable to DDT. We all have some of the stuff inside us and we always will (because it is stored in our fat), but not enough to matter. The argument of the opposition is that it is dangerous to meddle with the unknown. Since DDT is persistent, those small amounts are cumulative, adding up over the years, and there may come a time when they will matter. Man is at the top of the food chain (that is, we eat animals which have eaten other forms of life which have eaten pests killed by DDT); the more the stuff is spread around the more likely it is to affect our health eventually. But at the moment it looks as if the use of pesticides is coming under official control, though not to the extent many people would like. DDT has been banned in the USA, and a battle of doctors versus ecologists has started. The doctors say DDT is needed for killing insects, such as mosquitoes, which carry disease (quite different from crop spraying) and for killing moths which are attacking forests. The ecologists say the moths have only increased to danger point because birds which normally kept their numbers down have been killed by DDT. And so the argument goes on. . . .

There's not much we can do about it except to get unsprayed produce, but only a small fraction of it is guaranteed. Fish gulp all sorts of chemicals which get into rivers and sea, bees may collect honey from sprayed flowers, free-range hens may swallow the wrong grubs, and beef cattle may be contaminated in pastures treated with herbicides to kill off the weeds. So bar moving to a private island, the urban housewife has very little freedom of choice in these matters.

In the matter of additives, however, the outlook is somewhat brighter. If people feel strongly enough, they can influence industry. But as it is there are two groups—those who couldn't care less what is in the food they buy, and those who have been stirred up by alarmists but have insufficient knowledge to argue with officialdom.

Food reformers complain that during refining a vital part of food is removed and then, to add insult to injury, other synthetic substances are added as preservatives, flavourings, colourings or improvers. These additives may possibly be harmful in themselves or, more likely, may combine with other components to form harmful compounds—we just don't know. As it is, only single additives are tested.

Oddly enough, more orthodox people are worried about this

aspect of food processing than about alleged deficiencies. Concern about the unknown effects of additives is justified by the following rather startling facts:

1. There are more than one thousand additives, three-quarters of them synthetic, in common use. Flavourings comprise the largest group.
2. All *new* additives must be tested, but most of the older ones are still around. It is hoped to test everything eventually, but with present facilities and backlog it will take a long time.
3. A test of a single substance takes two to five years (because successive generations of animals are involved) and costs around $100,000. Only a few laboratories are equipped to perform the tests, and these laboratories are booked up for tests for years to come, with present facilities.

The attitude of officialdom is "Don't fuss. Just don't listen to alarmists; everything is under control; all additives will have to be tested eventually; of course no poisons are allowed." Why then do some things slip through and only get banned after years of use, such as butter yellow, agene (predecessor of chlorine dioxide in bread) and cyclamates? The answer given is that the ban errs on the safe side. For example agene was proved (after thirty years of argument) to be a nerve poison in the case of dogs. This does not mean it would do humans any harm, but the possibility was accepted. In the USA there is a section of the food regulations known as the Delaney Clause, which states that any substance which proves carcinogenic to an animal in any dose and under any conditions, must be banned. Many scientists feel that a large dose injected under the skin is quite different from a small dose taken by mouth. But since the skin injection caused tumours in mice, cyclamates were banned, and many other countries followed suit.

Has chlorine dioxide, objected to by food reformers, been tested? Yes, but no positive conclusions have been reached.

More tests are needed. Meanwhile it is taking its place in the line. (Food reformers think that chlorine dioxide, by destroying vitamin E, affects EFA. The Stanton/Price theory (Chapter V) suggests that it contributes to atherosclerosis.)

What happens when an additive comes under suspicion? Is it banned? Not necessarily. Results seem to vary. If the critics are in the minority, the complaint simply gets lost, as with chlorine dioxide. Sometimes the additive is given a temporary lease of life pending further tests. Or, if the additive performs a definitely useful service it may be allowed to continue until a safer substitute can be found. This is the case with nitrites, used as a preservative and to give a pink colour in cured meats. Nitrites sometimes combine with amines from amino acids to produce nitrosamines in the stomach. Nitrosamines in high concentration have been shown to produce cancer in animals, though no harm has been reported in humans. Since botulism (what you get if the meat goes bad) is deadly, it is thought that the devil you know is better than the devil you don't know. Plenty of people have died of botulism. Nobody has died of cancer caused by nitrosamines—as far as we know. Besides the cancer threat, the claim that nitrites destroy EFA seems a minor snag though probably more real.

Preservatives are the most necessary of the additives. It is colourings, flavourings, and improvers that seem unnecessary. But since nothing definite has been proved against them, we accept them. We, the human guinea pigs, have not been living with additives long enough yet for any long-term effects to show. Few people read the list of ingredients on a can or package, and even if they did, they would not object.

Those who are still worried about the situation can avoid additives by cutting out everything packaged, canned, bottled or processed except possibly some (though not all) products of health food shops. And they would also have to think twice about the origin of their meat, since livestock have been drawn into the clever chemistry business.

It has been found that two things can speed growth (and increase profits) in animals—antibiotics and hormones.

Antibiotics work by reducing the parasite population in the gut, particularly in poultry. The antibiotic is added to the feed. Any residue in the meat is destroyed by cooking.

Hormones work as chemical castrators and hence allow extra plumpness (as in capons). The hormone is administered as a pellet in the neck of a chicken or the ear of a calf. These are cut off before the meat is sold, but worriers think they are added to feeds and so get back into another lot of meat.

In 1960 it was discovered that bacteria which have become resistant to certain antibiotics can transmit their resistance to other bacteria of the same strain. This means that by eating meat containing immune bacteria, one can immunise the bacteria normally resident in the intestine, and these could transmit their resistance to a disease germ of the same strain, such as typhoid. The typhoid would then be resistant to penicillin or other therapeutic drugs which had been used on the animals.

As well as additives in food, we have additives in water—chlorine universally and fluorine in a few areas. Chlorine protects against bacteria and is acknowledged as an essential hygienic precaution. Those who think chlorine harmful don't get much of a hearing—again, probably, because the devil you know is better than the devil you don't know. Chlorine is said to destroy vitamin E and consequently to affect EFA. According to the Stanton/Price theory it increases cholesterol deposits. If lack of vitamin E causes EFA to be oxidised, leaving cholesterol without a partner, this seems a logical argument. Boiling all drinking water is the answer, says Dr Stanton.

Fluorine is added to water by certain local authorities, not all, as sodium fluroride, which in the proportion of one part per million, protects teeth. Above 7 ppm it is thought to be harmful. It has been suggested that the level of fluoride which is necessary in preventing cavities is dangerously close to the level which produces harmful results. A naturopath describes fluoridation as "the biggest hoax in medical history". Several European countries have now banned the practice. What are the snags? Apart from mottling teeth if the concentration is too high, fluorine is thought to inhibit the action of enzymes which are essential to metabolism, and to interfere with calcium deposition. The El Molo tribe in Kenya, who live beside a lake with high fluorine content, all have deformed bones. Reformers say that fluoridation tackles the problem of tooth decay from the wrong end. While consumption of soft drinks remains so high, other measures are futile.

The first two categories of poisons, concerning the composition of the food in the stores, are under the control of food producers and manufacturers and the Food and Drug Administration. The third category—what we decide to eat—is under our own control and for this reason is of more interest to the individual.

There are many food reformers who are convinced that most disease is caused by toxaemia brought about by the habitual eating of the wrong foods over the years. Does that mean that illness will only show up in the middle-aged and elderly? No, say investigators; certain diseases of children are a legacy from the mother—not genetically inherited but passed on to the developing child by the mother's toxic bloodstream.

The idea behind all this is simple. We need certain nutrients for provision of energy and for body building and repair. (See Chapter II.) These nutrients are taken in food, digested, assimilated, and sent via the bloodstream to the cells which need them. Here they are processed and used to perform different functions. The waste products of metabolism are returned to the blood and sent to the organs of elimination—the lungs, kidneys and skin. Provided the food contains nutrients in the normal proportions needed by the body, the business of metabolism will proceed smoothly and the body will be healthy. But if the nutrients are taken in the wrong proportions over a long period, together with substances that the body does not want at all, then trouble starts. There will be more waste products than the body is designed to deal with. They may be eliminated successfully for a time, but gradually they will accumulate and "gum up the works". It may be many years before any recognisable disease occurs, but sooner or later it will. Disease, in fact, is the body's attempt to get rid of poisonous wastes. (Fever, by increasing metabolic rate, speeds elimination.)

This is, of course, the Nature Cure theory, but it is also supported by a small minority of qualified doctors. Of these, Dr H. G. Bieler of California has set out the idea in most detail in his book *Food Is Your Best Medicine.*

Dr Bieler, a keen mountaineer in his seventies, tells us that his philosophy developed as a result of personal illness as a young, overworked GP. Although trained in the use of drugs as the basis of treatment, he decided to study diet and before long had cured himself. He continued to study, did much experimental and laboratory work and, convinced that he was on the right track, applied the diet theories to his patients. For fifty years this was so successful that Dr Bieler found himself unable to retire—patients continued to track him down. Although the idea of replacing drugs by foods is not accepted with much enthusiasm by orthodox medicine, Dr Bieler has never fallen foul of his more conventional colleagues; in fact a chair of Dietetic Medicine at Columbia University (the Tilden-Weger-Bieler Chair) has been named for him in conjunction with two other pioneers.

Expanding the Nature Cure theory, Dr Bieler suggests that the body has three lines of defence against toxaemia:

1. The first is the digestive tract. If the food eaten is poisonous enough, it will be rejected by vomiting or diarrhoea.
2. If the food is somewhat less toxic, or the poison is more diluted, it will be absorbed then dealt with by the liver, the second line of defence. Either the toxin will be neutralised or it will be sent back to the intestine via the bile. Provided the liver is efficient, the bloodstream will remain pure, though the bile will be corrosive, possibly causing a bilious attack.
3. If the liver is unable to deal with the poison, it will enter

the bloodstream and possibly damage the kidneys which are only designed to eliminate normal by-products of metabolism. When there is more toxic material in the bloodstream than can be dealt with by the organs of elimination, "emergency vicarious elimination" comes into play—the lungs try to help out the kidneys, the skin takes over from the liver and, as a last resort, the endocrine glands, the third line of defence, join in the struggle. This is a new extension of the toxaemia theory, but one which explains pretty nearly all diseases. For example when the lungs are involved we get bronchitis, pneumonia and TB. When the skin is involved we get skin diseases, dandruff and catarrh; when the glands are involved we get migraine or epilepsy (from swelling of the pituitary), arthritis, catarrh or appendicitis (from inflammation of the middle and inner skins which are affected by thyroid activity) and fever or cancer due to over-activity of the adrenal glands.

According to Dr Bieler, the causes of toxaemia are: Excess acid (from too much starch or protein).
Stimulating foods, particularly tea, coffee and condiments.
Pharmaceutical drugs.
Artificial foods, including synthetic additives. The very fact that they are not found in nature makes them unacceptable to the system.

The treatment of mild cases consists of fasting, then gradually neutralising the poison, usually by means of alkaline vegetables. In severe cases the cure must be supervised, since any sudden change of diet may cause alarming symptoms.

Though many writers murmur vaguely about the evils of alcohol, tea, coffee, salt, vinegar and strong seasonings, the whys and wherefores are rarely explained. Being unconvinced, addicts continue to take their favourite tipple with a clear conscience. Dr Bieler, however, does not let us off. He explains that tea, coffee and table salt are stimulants. They whip the adrenal glands into activity, which, we may remember, has the effect of preparing the body for fight and flight. Sugar is poured into the bloodstream, blood pressure is raised, and one feels a surge of energy and well-being. It is this energy-producing effect which makes us addicts without realising it. But taking stimulants, even mild, everyday ones, is about as sensible as whipping an exhausted horse to make it go faster. It will—until it collapses.

Unlike many food reform writers, who lay down specific "cures" for the world in general, Dr Bieler stresses that no two cases are alike, "one man's meat is another man's poison", and any treatment must be tailored to the dietary history and chemical make-up of the individual.

Having heard the case against processed foods from the poison and deficiency angles, let us see what health foods have to offer.

D I A L O G U E

Q. *What effect is DDT thought to have, by those who object to its use?*
A. DDT is a nerve poison, killing insects by destroying the nervous system. In larger animals it is known to interfere with oxidation and also to stimulate the activity of enzymes which destroy oestrogens. Birds affected in this way either fail to breed, or lay soft-shelled eggs which break easily. DDT is also thought to cause liver damage. Though most doctors say no ill effects have ever been reported in humans, (not even those associated with the manufacture or use of DDT sprays) there are others who say DDT poisoning does exist. The difficulty lies in establishing cause and effect.

Q. *Is there any alternative to DDT?*
A. The organo-phosphates (as opposed to organo-chlorides like DDT and its derivatives) are less persistent but even more deadly while they last. Users have to take more care and in some cases need protective clothing. A new development is

systemics which poison predators from inside the plant. Applied to the soil, they enter the sap, protect the plant during growth, then decompose when the vulnerable stage is past. Needless to say, there are people who suspect the whole business and regard this as the unkindest cut of all. Meanwhile research on biological control continues, but not fast enough for an expanding world population and its need for food.

Q. *Is not the outcry about additives rather alarmist, bearing in mind official interest in safety and welfare?*
A. The outcry, from a comparatively small minority, is often without any scientific basis except the rather astonishing figures quoted previously. These numbers sound rather overwhelming and naturally give rise to questions, but there is no reason to assume that all additives are a menace to health. How many of the total are we likely to eat? On an average diet, maybe twenty a day—bread alone contains up to a dozen. Two points concern worriers—first the length of time taken to settle the matter when there is a doubt, and secondly the number of items banned by other countries which are allowed here.

To illustrate the first point, we may note, dragging in agene again, that it took nearly thirty years of argument before it was finally banned. Agene's successor, chlorine dioxide, is now suspect, but no definite decision has been reached after nearly twenty years. But if chlorine destroys vitamin E in the body (there's not much left in bread) leaving EFA unprotected, it seems logical to assume that the EFA will be oxidised by chlorine dioxide, which is above all an oxidising agent.

Synthetic anti-oxidants are another example. Suspected about fifteen years ago, they have been banned then reinstated. Now allowed in limited quantities in certain foods, they are still regarded as harmful by many scientists.

While the truth about additives is practically impossible to evaluate, that oft-heard bromide "no apparent adverse effect" comforts most people. The more emotional of the back to nature folk continue to rail against 'chemicals' without quite knowing why. It remains for the more scientific of the protesters to put it into words—our system has been evolved to deal with compounds occurring in living foods; we have enzymes to digest and process these substances. But synthetic compounds cannot be dealt with by the body. Unless neutralised or eliminated they will accumulate as poisons. However, we are not completely defenceless—the liver is designed to deal with a limited amount of poison.

Q. *Are not the quantities involved in additives too small to be poisonous?*
A. Not much is known about micro-chemistry as yet, which is why there is a certain amount of anxiety. But it seems as though very small quantities of a substance can have important effects both good and bad. We already know of several examples in this category:

> The doses effective in homoeopathy, which are minute.
> The one part per million of fluoride which is thought to protect teeth.
> The trace elements already known, which are essential to life in doses too small to measure.
> Hundreds of acres of tomato plants were mysteriously killed off in Great Britain some years ago. It was only after prolonged investigation that the trouble was traced to residue from a pesticide factory, which got into a river in quantities too small to be measured by normal methods In the USA chicks were killed by a pesticide residue diluted to one part in 20 million.

There are three unknown factors about additives—their direct effect, their effect in conjunction with other substances, which might be synergistic, and their possible cumulative effect.

Q. *What about alleged mistakes in eating?*
A. These come under two headings: things which we shouldn't eat at all (according to food reformers), and good foods eaten to excess. The first group comprises "the four whites", i.e. white sugar, white bread, white rice and salt, and stimulants.

1. The case against white sugar has been explained in detail in Chapter V. However, if you decide to give it up, you want to be able to say exactly why, so here is a brief summary of what food reformers think about it:

    a. It is too concentrated, which means one tends to take too much. Apart from the obvious increase in weight, hormone balance may be affected; extra insulin is called for, and this may eventually upset hormone balance in general.

    b. Sugar lacks vitamin B, needed in the metabolism of carbohydrates, so either existing supplies are drawn on and depleted, or sugar is left partly processed, in a poisonous form.

    c. Sugar is what reformers call a foodless food, meaning that the nutrients which accompany carbohydrates in their natural state are missing. We feel hunger for energy foods, not for nutrients. In nature both go together. But if hunger is satisfied by the energy value of sugar, malnutrition may result.

    d. Sugar is acid forming, and we already have an over-acid diet. Fruit cooked or eaten with sugar becomes acid, so the benefit of its original alkaline reaction is lost.

    e. Sugar, particularly in soft drinks, causes tooth decay.

    f. Sugar may encourage production of cholesterol, either on its own or in combination with fats.

    g. Sugar may aggravate indigestion and ulcers.

Figures show that the consumption of sugar has gone *slightly* down since 1970 in Britain, Switzerland, and Australia. This is probably more in the interests of dieting than due to any belief that sugar is a "poison", but the trend has prompted some hilarious advertising from the Sugar Information Bureau in New York:

Surprise! Sugar isn't a bad guy. The sugar in a soft drink or ice cream cone, shortly before mealtime, turns into energy fast. And that energy could be just the energy you need to say no to those extra helpings. That's why sugar is a good guy. Surprise! . . . only eighteen calories per teaspoon, and it's all energy.

2. White bread versus brown is the subject of such heated debate that the main points can bear summarising again. Is white bread a passport to disease? Food reformers say:

a. The lack of fibre is the most serious thing, leading to constipation and after many years perhaps diverticular disease, varicose veins and other ailments not usually connected with diet. But you can, of course, get your fibre in some other form (bran by the bag, or vegetable fibre) while continuing to eat white bread. Eating germ bread won't help the fibre problem.

b. The authors of *The Saccharine Disease* suggest that the reduced protein content of white bread has a connection with ulcers, and that the concentration, though much less than that of sugar, might contribute to obesity and diabetes.

c. Many valuable ingredients are lost during refining—the germ, and a number of vitamins and minerals. These can be made up from other foods provided one makes the effort. But those who eat out, dislike salads, and fill up on snacks and convenience foods might miss out.

d. As with sugar, it is easy to satisfy hunger by eating too much white bread, crowding out more valuable foods.

e. Chlorine dioxide, which bleaches and improves, is thought to destroy vitamin E, leaving EFA unprotected. According to the Stanton/Price theory (Chapter V) the chlorine combines with cholesterol to form deposits in the arteries.

If you believe this last claim, then white bread is a passport to disease. If you don't, then the verdict seems to be—white bread is an inferior food, but its shortcomings can be offset by a careful choice of diet.

3. White rice comes somewhere between sugar and white bread as a "non-food", but since it is eaten comparatively rarely in this country its shortcomings are less important. Parboiled rice has some vitamin B diffused through the grain, so it is a better food than ordinary polished rice.

4. Salt is the subject of universal agreement among nutritionists, orthodox and otherwise. Nobody (except possibly those recipe writers who say "add salt and pepper to taste") has a good word to say for it. We need salt, but ample exists in foods. The extra we add in cooking and at the table gives us ten times more than we need. Vast amounts are added to canned and processed foods, on account of salt's preservative qualities. Since salt eating is an addiction, you feel terrible if you suddenly try to do without it. But once adapted (according to the Stefansson legend) everything is fine. The evils of salt are said to be:

a. By increasing water retention, particularly in blood fluid, salt raises blood pressure.
b. It forms deposits which cause hardening of the arteries.
c. By interfering with uric acid excretion, salt aggravates rheumatism and arthritis.
d. Taken over a long period, salt causes a strain on the kidneys and possible eventual damage.
e. Salt is thought to displace calcium, which maybe the basis of the saying "salt is bad for your nerves".

As long as the kidneys are healthy, surplus salt is eliminated, but over the years they may lose their efficiency and salt is retained, with adverse effects.

5. Having disposed of the four whites, of which sugar and salt seem to be the ones to take most seriously, we come to stimulants. These inclue tea, coffee, alcohol, cola, condiments, vinegar and strong spices. Why are we told to do

without some of the best things in food and drink? What does a stimulant do and how can it be bad for one?

As we saw in Chapter II a stimulant speeds up metabolism in readiness for some extra effort. Blood vessels contract, blood pressure goes slightly up, sugar is released into the blood and the kidneys are prodded into action to clear the bloodstream of wastes. The result is a temporary feeling of warmth and well-being, followed by a let-down. Provided the stimulation is moderate, the let-down passes unnoticed. But excessive dependence on say, tea or coffee sets up a vicious cycle, since the ensuing depression soon gives rise to a desire for more. We then get the picture of a person unable to work without a succession of cups of something, plus cigarettes. It is the perpetual overworking of the kidneys leading to eventual damage, which is the most serious outcome of the stimulation habit, say food reformers.

Caffeine, the stimulant in tea and coffee, is also a purine, a substance which increases the formation of uric acid. Hence the connection between the perpetual cup of tea and rheumatism. Then there is the news that tea contains quite a lot of fluorine. Altogether, coffee (or tea) breaks seem to be less of a blessing than we thought.

This brings us to the final poison category—good foods eaten in the wrong proportions. Imbalance of nutrients, say some food reformers, can lead to corresponding imbalance of the "friendly and unfriendly" bacteria in the colon. The former synthesise vitamins B and K, the latter cause putrefaction, creating toxins which may be re-absorbed. Excess protein or refined carbohydrate and lack of fibre may throw the balance out. But this is only one aspect of imbalance.

The good foods most likely to be eaten to excess are proteins and fats. Fats in their natural state are probably self-limiting, since too much becomes nauseating. It is more likely to be hidden fats in cakes, biscuits, pastry and ice cream, which are over-consumed. An article in the *British Medical Journal* points out that the term "vegetable oil", assumed by those innocent shoppers who actually read labels, to be unsaturated, may be a cover-up for the worst fat of the lot—coconut. It is 85 per cent saturated and contains palmitic acid, "a potent atherogenic agent". "A deplorable commercial secrecy envelops the topic of edible fats," states the article. "We consume commercially processed foods without considering what they contain, how they are made or what harm they do." Excess saturated fat, as we have seen, increases blood cholesterol and so leads to possible atherosclerosis. And excess PUFA, according to some investigators, has its own dangers if unaccompanied by adequate vitamin E (Chapter V).

Is excess protein a poison? Many food reformers think so. (See also Chapter III.) Dr Bieler, in his chapter "Proteins can be body killers" sums up the situation like this:

1. Protein is essential for growth and development. The amount needed can be assessed from the amount in mother's milk. Human milk has the lowest protein content of any mammal because the human baby grows more slowly than other mammals.

2. After growth is completed, the amount of protein needed is that required to maintain nitrogen equilibrium, but most of us eat far more than this. Excess puts a strain on liver (which breaks protein down) and kidneys (which have to eliminate the excess). This may be tolerated for a time, but with increasing age both liver and kidneys fail and toxaemia builds up. Some proteins, which are also purines, produce uric acid.

3. When protein is cooked, its structure is changed to a less digestible form and putrefactive acids are formed. In small amounts these can be neutralised by a healthy liver, and eliminated via the bile. In excess, or with a weakened liver, they cannot. The diseases most associated with excess protein, Dr Bieler thinks, are polio in young people and cancer in older groups. (An experiment has linked polio with ice cream, made from heated, pasteurised milk. Experiments with cats proved that cats fed on

cooked meat and milk products became sick, developed degenerative diseases and died early.) Primitive people such as Australian aborigines, Eskimos and Alaskan Indians living on raw meat and fish were examples of perfect health before they took to a civilised diet. The explorer Stefansson and his assistants lived on raw meat in the Arctic but suffered indigestion when they cooked the meat.

A person who eats a lot of cooked meat, therefore, has to cope with poisons of three different origins:

   a. Urea and uric acid, the normal end products of protein. Eliminated by healthy kidneys.
   b. Poisons made by bacteria which get to work on flesh as soon as an animal is killed. Dealt with by a healthy liver.
   c. Extra poisons (putrefactive acids) caused by alteration of the protein molecule during cooking. Dealt with by liver and kidneys until they become exhausted. Plenty of alkaline vegetables help.

Since raw meat is not popular (and probably unhygienic), Dr Bieler recommends lightly cooked meat, raw milk and eggs, nuts and vegetable proteins.

Q. *Why do so many high protein eaters enjoy excellent health?*
A. According to Dr Bieler, because they eat it raw, like the Australian aborigines, Eskimos and African pastoral tribes such as the Masai, who eat raw milk and blood. The healthy meat eaters in affluent societies are not really healthy at all, Dr Bieler claims. They appear so because of the stimulating effect of meat. But even while they are feeling so good, toxaemia may be building up. A wild theory? Maybe, but it was going around long before Adelle Davis, high protein advocate, died of cancer.

Q. *What is so terrible about frying?*

A. The snags are said to be:
1. Frying usually involves the use of saturated fat, which when burnt contains acrolein, a poison.
2. If an unsaturated fat is used, the vitamin E is lost and prolonged frying may turn the fat rancid. This is particularly likely if the same fat is used over again.

CHAPTER VIII

WHAT HEALTH FOODS HAVE TO OFFER

PEOPLE ARE EITHER suckers or cynics. Either you are completely sold on the health food idea or you read about it in the spirit of someone who goes to a fortune-teller—90 per cent for a laugh and 10 per cent because there just might be something in it.

That 10 per cent of the cynic which is open to conviction is very easily put off by wild exaggeration, and health food people are inclined to overstate their case and so weaken it. "The whiter the bread, the sooner you're dead" is a case in point. The man in the street can see plenty of white bread eaters who are far from dead, so he dismisses the whole idea as a lot of rubbish. "White sugar should be banned as the drug heroin is banned" is another wild statement which snuffs out the first glimmer of interest on the part of the waverer. We may agree that sugar eating is a form of addiction, that it is bad for you and may in time lead to obesity, diabetes or heart disease, but to compare it to a hard drug only weakens the argument.

Food reformers, in their efforts to condemn modern foods, are apt to get starry-eyed about the past. Our ancestors, they say, with their whole foods, were the picture of health. But were they? One of the qualities perfect health is supposed to impart is resistance to disease. In fact, according to Nature Cure, if you eat their way you can walk through a cholera epidemic and just snap your fingers at the bugs. But our ancestors couldn't. Healthy life or no, they died like flies from plague, smallpox, pneumonia, dysentery and tuberculosis.

Some food reformers are also starry-eyed about primitive people whose natural instincts are said to have led them to the right foods. But primitive people did not increase in numbers until modern medicine came along. Before that, most of them were riddled with malaria, yaws, sleeping sickness, bilharzia and other diseases.

But, say enthusiasts, these arguments can be answered. Our ancestors were divided into classes—the rich who over-ate, the poor who just didn't get enough, and a small section in the middle, which ate moderately. When disaster, in the form of an epidemic, struck, the top and bottom classes would be decimated but the ones in the middle would survive. The Black Death killed half the population of London, but in the absence of medical knowledge, this survival rate is quite high, so there must have been some tough people around. This is all the more remarkable when you realise that vitamin C, with its protective properties, was in short supply in the British diet in winter time until the widespread acceptance of potatoes in the eighteenth century.

As for primitive people, nobody is claiming that they know all the answers, only some of them. Their diseases, caused mainly by parasites which multiply in unhygienic conditions, were a form of population limitation, favouring survival of the healthy, or wise eaters. Only since these diseases have been controlled, have their populations increased. Before that, some of them may have stumbled on the right answers, or maybe worked them out by trial and error over generations. Those who didn't do so suffered. Protagonists of organic farming would say it's not what you eat but the way that you grow it that counts, and those primitive people who have stumbled on the fundamentals of the ecological cycle are the healthy ones.

Our departure from the simple life has led to the health food movement. But what are health foods? Many definitions have been given, perhaps the silliest being "food sold in a health food store". Ponderous and equally vague is the description "substances whose consumption is advocated by various health movements" (both from scientists, believe it or not). If we want to sum up what food reformers are aiming at it is simpler to say "natural foods with nothing added and nothing taken away".

The thing which seems to upset opponents of health food most is that it is big business. People who normally admire material success grow positively purple in the face when confronted with the business side of the growing health food movement. They point out that some supermarkets have health food sections, that some health food stores have been opened by tobacco interests or as part of the diversification programme of other large concerns. The critics are not so much worried that these shops may not know enough about the subject to sell the right things, but are indignant that money is being made at all. They point out that the health food trade accounts for millions of dollars a year, but fail to point out that this is only a small percentage of the total food profits.

The trouble seems to be that anything "good" is not supposed to be a commercial success, which is why clergymen come somewhere near the bottom of the pay scale. In 1970 a very amusing article appeared entitled "The Natural Goodness Business". The eye-catching introduction gave us a hint of what was to come. "In this wicked world one way to make money is by selling virtue—at very high prices."

The article rated 100 per cent for entertainment value but in common with many de-bunking articles its weapon was derision—the easiest weapon in the world to use. It concentrated on the sillier and crankier aspects of health foods (of which there are plenty), on the personal rivalries within the business (and what business is without them?) and on the fact that a whole chain of health food stores and manufacturers had been bought up by a firm of sugar importers.

But one range of products mentioned in the article was a line of tissue salts which could appear to encourage self-diagnosis by gullible hypochondriacs to a farcical degree. You name it—a twinge, a sniffle, a pimple—and there was a tissue salt to set you right. One in particular, for "watery symptoms", was plain salt, of which we already take ten times too much. This, I thought, was going altogether too far, for although the gullible may to some extent deserve what they get, surely it must take a fiend in human shape to so exploit the simple desire to feel well.

So it was with considerable surprise that I discovered the founder of the firm in question to be a kindly vegetarian Quaker, Mr Wallace Stocks, who practised what he preached and died only recently at the age of ninety-five. The idea resulted from the activities of Mr Stocks's uncle, apparently also kindly, who ran a business in India, became concerned about the poor health of his employees, and decided to try the new therapy on them. The results, we are told, were so spectacular that Mr Stocks decided his life work was to be the making and selling of the little pills, which contain only one part in a million of the salt that does the trick.

A somewhat more belligerent article appeared in the British magazine *Nova* ("So do you really need health food?" February 1973). This article was not enlivened by humour but aimed straight at the crookery angle: "What is a matter for concern is that an industry is mushrooming on the basis of exploiting vaguely defined anxieties about general health, and this industry is insufficiently examined, accountable or challenged." The implication clearly is that examining, accounting and challenging would reveal something pretty nasty in the wood-shed. Maybe a challenge of the patent medicine business or the colossal cosmetics industry might reveal a few skeletons under the floor-boards as well.

Then we come to the criticism that item by item, health foods are more expensive than "ordinary" foods, the implication being that some wicked ogre is taking advantage of the innocent seeker after health. What escapes notice is that health foods are as yet minority products and therefore cannot compete with mass production, also they are by their very nature more expensive to produce—the whole foods with their shorter shelf life, and the organically grown vegetables with their greater labour requirements.

Anyone who was utterly convinced that health foods mean better health and longer life would pay the extra price willingly. Just as Faust sold his soul to the devil for eternal life so we would sell the car and the TV for a few more healthy years if we were absolutely certain. But are health foods really all they're cracked up to be, or is the whole thing a delusion if not actually a racket?

Before we try to answer this question, let's summarise the main ways in which food reformers feel our diet falls short of the ideal, and the ways in which health foods claim to put it right. Sticking to poisons and deficiencies we get the following:

Possible poisons in or resulting from modern diet	Food Reform Solution	Health Food
Additives (improvers, preservatives, colours, flavourings).	Unadulterated food	Stone-ground flour, bran bread, granolo, peanut butter, dairy produce from approved farms, pure honey. NB Some health food manufacturers accept sulphur dioxide.
Antibiotics in meat or poultry Hormones in meat or poultry	Avoid products of commercial farming	Free range eggs and poultry Textured soya meat
Residue from pesticides or herbicides	Organically grown produce	Organically grown fruit and vegetables
Toxic residues from meat	Restrict protein to 10 per cent of calories, greater emphasis on vegetable protein	Nuts, dried beans, soya meat, unprocessed cheese
Acid system due to excess acid-forming foods	Eat more fruit and vegetables (alkaline) and milk (neutral)	Organically grown fruit and vegetables
Alcohol		Juice bar, bottled juices

Possible poisons in or resulting from modern diet	Food Reform Solution	Health Food
Sugar (Refined)	Get sweet flavours from fruit or honey in moderation	Brown sugar (called "raw"), fresh fruit, dried fruit free from sulphur and mineral oil, molasses, carob (a sweet bean), honey
Table salt	Avoid excess	Sea salt (contains other minerals said to balance harmful effects of sodium chloride), vegetable salt, kelp
Caffeine and tannin	As above	Herb teas, decaffeinated coffee

*   *   *

Possible Deficiency	Remarks	Health Food
Vitamin A	Deficiency unlikely with balanced diet	Carrot juice (via carotene) Supplements (fish oil)
B	Water soluble. Needed daily	Wholemeal bread and flour, wheat germ, brown rice, soya products, yeast, yoghurt, supplements
C	Water soluble. Needed daily	Juices, fruit and vegetables, supplements
D	Deficiency unlikely in adults except the elderly	Soft margarine, supplements
E	No agreement on requirements	Sunflower seeds, wheat germ supplements
F (EFA)	Important to take extra vitamin E with oils	Vegetable oil or soft margarine
P	Usually associated with C	Whole fruits (not juices), supplements

Possible Deficiency	Remarks	Health Food
Lecithin	Thought to emulsify cholesterol	Granules or capsules
Calcium	Added to all bread except wholewheat	Cheese, yoghurt, kelp, supplements
Iron	Should not be taken on do-it-yourself basis or within twelve hours of taking Vitamin E which it destroys	Organically grown produce, molasses
Potassium	Most likely to be deficient in eaters of convenience foods	Organically grown produce, honey, molasses, kelp, apple cider vinegar
Magnesium	Occurs in all greens Deficiency unlikely	With calcium in dolomite tablets
Trace minerals	Important as constituents of enzymes and for treatment of arthritis	Organically grown produce, herbs, kelp, elixirs
Other minerals		Supplements, herbs, kelp, elixirs, "tissue salts"
Fibre		Bran bread, bran by the bag, fruit and vegetables

From this we can see that the Health Food Store sells a lot besides food. At least half its trade is in pills and tablets and there is a pretty good line in herbal remedies, the "natural" branch of the patent medicine business. The latest departure is natural cosmetics.

The bottled side of the business is pretty fair game for the sniper whether he is a doctor reiterating that we get our vitamins with knife and fork, or a normal, well-balanced reporter who likes to take a crack at anything that savours of the eccentric, the mystical and the slightly nutty.

Pills, mainly vitamin and mineral supplements, appeal to those who want to keep fit without doing too much calculating of nutritional values every time they go shopping. It's the short-cut, magic-cure-all outlook which we discussed in Chapter I, and though the vitamin may be from natural rather than synthetic sources, this solution is not supported by Nature Cure, the organic farming people, or anyone who believes that nature knows best. Supplements are supported to some extent by the schools of nutrition represented by Gayelord Hauser, Lelord Kordel, J. I. Rodale (all three have their own range of supplements) and Adelle Davis. Their view is that nutrition has got into such a mess that no one living in the concrete jungle has a hope of a reasonable diet without supplements. They deplore the situation, but there it is. As long as there are people who prefer short cuts, and as long as organically grown produce is in short supply (and some of it at least is phoney), this may be a realistic view.

The skulduggery aspect of health food is the final target of its opponents. *Time* magazine recounts the story of a farmer who sprayed his crops by night then sold them as free of pesticides. *Prevention*'s editor puts the proportion of phoney produce at 50 per cent to 70 per cent of all that is labelled "organic", and many other tales are told of sleight of hand twixt field and shop. In Britain, both the Soil Association and *The Organic Food Finder* (Rodale Press) award a symbol to approved producers which should ensure integrity, but the average shopper accepts a plain label which means nothing.

As well as vitamin and mineral pills, we have herb pills (though herbs are also sold dry, as flavourings and as teas) and elixirs. A few years ago the mention of herbs would conjure up visions of a lady in a smock knocking up pot-pourri or dandelion wine for the village fete. But now, with the back-to-nature movement, herbs and witch-doctor stunts are gaining new recognition.

The theory behind the herbal remedy is perfectly simple. There are various vitamins, minerals and compounds (including poisons) which do specific things, some good, some bad, in a pretty reliable way. These effects have been noticed over the ages by witch-doctors, Chinese sages, South American Indians, Papuan head-hunters and such, and the results handed down from generation to generation. Some of the less respectable witch-doctors (like their descendants, the phoney organic farmers) may have exploited their patients and so given witch-doctoring a bad name, but in many cases the old mumbo-jumbo cures have been found to have a logical basis. And just as we know that the vitamin content of vegetables varies according to the season, so the old witch doctors knew from experience that the potency of their herbs varied with the time of year.

The snag with herbs is that the active ingredients (if any) are not all scientifically understood, so their use is a matter of guesswork. So if you are hooked on the idea of herbs you fancy taking the lot, just to be on the safe side, and this is where elixirs come in. They contain hundreds of herbal extracts, and as with hundreds of anything, you have to pay accordingly. On the whole, dried herbs are great for flavouring, herb tea is quite pleasant, while the pills and potions appeal to those who like vague phrases such as "cleanses the system", "tones the liver", "purifies the blood", and have plenty of money to experiment with.

Perhaps the big advantage of herbs (in common with vegetables in general) is that they are sources of trace minerals, known and unknown, understood and otherwise. Since they take up only a small space, they can be grown by almost anyone. Some even grow wild.

Go into any health food store for the first time, and you may be surprised to see a number of items which can also be bought in the supermarket. What is the advantage of the health food version? Here are some answers given by health food manufacturers:

Item	Advantage of health food version
Yoghurt	Only a few farms supply health food yoghurt, which is made from raw certified milk with none of the ingredients destroyed by pasteur-

isation. No emulsifiers (often made from saturated fats) are added as is the case in commercial yoghurts. When fruit is added, this is the real thing with no synthetic flavouring.

Cheese

No superiority is claimed for health food cheese. It caters to the vegan market, being made with a vegetable rennet instead of the normal type from the stomach of a calf.

Ice cream

Commercial ice cream is a cooked product combining white sugar with saturated fat such as palm oil or coconut oil. Artificial flavourings and colourings may be used. Health food ice cream is made from raw milk, cream and natural flavouring.

Peanut butter

Commercial types are often hydrogenated and may contain sugar as well as too much salt. Homogenisers and emulsifiers are added to prevent a layer of oil from remaining on the top. Health food types may contain a vegetable stabiliser (from soya) for this purpose.

Dried fruit

That sold in health food stores is without sulphur dioxide and liquid paraffin.

Salad oils

Usually no difference. In theory cold-pressed oils should be available but in practice are hard to come by. Most health food stores sell branded types, identical to those in the supermarket.

Ceylon tea

Slightly lower in tannin, otherwise no difference.

Eggs

Free-range eggs have more EFA and less saturated fat than other eggs.

Salt   Health stores sell sea salt which contains small
                amounts of other minerals in addition to
                sodium chloride. Since the body fluid is similar
                to sea water, it is thought that the balance of
                minerals in sea salt is more acceptable to the
                body.

Honey   Most commercial honey is pasteurised to delay
                crystallisation. It is also heated to facilitate
                filtering. Filter-pressing is a specially efficient
                method which removes all the pollen as well as
                impurities. Health store honey is strained
                through a mesh which removes impurities but
                leaves the pollen in. "Creamed" honey, the
                least desirable of the commercial types, may
                contain commercial glucose (corn syrup)
                which is made from the action of acid on corn
                starch. It bears no relation to natural glucose
                (blood sugar) but because of its cheapness is
                added to many foods as a sweetener. It is even
                more rapidly absorbed than refined sugar.

DIALOGUE

Q. *What conditions are necessary for a store to call itself a
health food store?*
A. None. Any restaurant which serves a plate of wilting salad
can call itself a health food restaurant even though the shelves
are lined with cans and any shop or counter selling wheat
germ, yoghurt (any kind) and salad oil (any kind) plus some
pills and potions can carry a sign "Health Foods". Very often
patent medicines creep in, which is the very antithesis of the
health idea. The value of the store depends entirely on the
integrity of the proprietor.

Q. *Can one say that the food sold in health stores lives up to the definition "nothing added and nothing taken away"?*
A. The contents of the average health store can be divided roughly into a third wholefoods, a third pills, potions and cosmetics and a third packaged and convenience foods. This latter section is growing fast. It includes breakfast foods, mixes, soya meat products and food for dieters. Though mainly free from additives, the mixes represent a trend away from wholefoods. Some of the breakfast foods contain brown sugar and a small amount of preservative.

Among the pills and potions we can see a definite trend towards medicine. Originally, the pills were supplements, replacing nutrients lost in processing. Now there are indigestion cures, tranquillisers, reducing tablets, and rheumatism cures (mainly herbal).

We have to remember that the health food business is commercial, and though there is nothing wrong in making money by supplying a need, the general idea of a healthy diet tends to be obscured by the popular wish to cure aches and pains by means of some magic potion while continuing bad habits as before. You can, for instance, buy fructose or fruit sugar in a health shop. Since it is sweeter than sucrose you need less of it—but it is refined sugar all the same. You can also get nicotine-free cigarettes. But many people think the danger of a cigarette lies not only in the nicotine but in the high temperature at which the smoke enters the lungs.

Finally we come to the nonsense side of health foods. Though many who are not health nuts would agree that wholewheat bread and unadulterated foods might be a good idea, the cynic draws the line at pollen, ginseng and pumpkin seeds. In all fairness we must admit that pollen is undergoing trials in several hospitals and ginseng is being researched in Germany.

Q. *What is ginseng?*
A. A root which hails from Korea. When dried, powdered and eaten it is said to make a new person of you. Ginseng has been

doing this for people for several thousand years, which is why its proponents believe so firmly in it. It has stood the test of time, they say; if it wasn't any good, surely it would have dropped out of use by now? Perhaps the research now going on in Germany will tell us the answer.

Q. *What is kelp?*
A. A seaweed which, since it grows in the sea, contains a large number of minerals (sixty they say), including trace minerals. Since the role of trace minerals is not fully understood (we don't know which ones are needed for what) and they are said to be less available than formerly in the soil, taking kelp is a good way of making sure of your quota. This is thought to be particularly important in the case of arthritis.

Q. *Is health store bread made from compost-grown wheat?*
A. Some is, some isn't. There is not enough compost-grown wheat to supply demand. The main health advantage of health store bread is retention of all the bran (which makes it somewhat solid) and freedom from additives. Germ bread, being made from white flour plus germ, cannot make the claim "nothing added, nothing taken away".

Q. *Why is processed cheese generally played down by health food people?*
A. Processed cheese is ordinary cheese which has been melted down, pasteurised, and had flavour and emulsifier added before repacking. Processing gives a new lease on life to cheese which would otherwise have passed its peak flavour. So it is less "natural" than ordinary cheese.

Q. *What is so great about molasses?*
A. It was one of Gayelord Hauser's original wonder foods and his alternative to refined sugar. It is the residue left behind during sugar refining, retaining various vitamins and minerals, particularly potassium. But it is still a very concentrated

food, no good for sweetening and definitely an acquired taste. You can get the minerals from fruit, vegetables and kelp without going through the agony of eating molasses.

Q. *What is the great reputation of honey based on?*
A. Honey, like ginseng, has been popular for thousands of years, and this fact is often quoted in support of its virtues. But honey was for thousands of years the only concentrated sweetener—sugar came along a mere four hundred years ago—so its long-standing popularity is easily accounted for. Is honey superior to sugar? It contains vitamins and minerals in small quantities (not enough to make much contribution to diet) though the trace minerals and waxes, which have not yet been studied, might be important. But honey is almost as concentrated as sugar, it enters the bloodstream faster, it is just as fattening in excess and just as dangerous to diabetics and heart cases, say experts, though because of its strong flavour it is difficult to eat so much. Honey's supporters often mention its speed of absorption as an advantage. But though this might be useful in an emergency, as part of a normal diet, rapid absorption is not a virtue but a vice. (See Chapter V.)

On the other side of the coin we have many stories of wounds healing and sick people being cured with honey. Enthusiasts often claim that their pet food is eaten by long-living people. So we find claims that the famous Georgian centenarians are beekeepers. Others say they eat yoghurt, and pollen fans say they eat pollen. Perhaps they eat the lot.

Q. *What is so special about cider vinegar?*
A. Nobody knows. Cider vinegar with honey was the special hobby horse of Dr Jarvis, author of the best-selling books *Vermont Folk Medicine* and *Arthritis and Folk Medicine*. People who tried the mixture raved about it. Whole industries were founded on the strength of its popularity, and 'Honegar', for those too lazy to mix their own juice, still sells. But read the books and you are faced with a puzzle, for Dr Jarvis's views are the opposite of everybody else's. While most views

say we need more alkaline food, Jarvis says we need more acid. The general view is that protein is acid-forming. Jarvis says it is alkaline. He thinks the tissues are encrusted like a kettle with the calcium precipitated from hard water (Vermont is a limestone area) and this needs to be dissolved in an acid such as vinegar—an odd view for a qualified medical man to hold. But it seems that the views, odd or otherwise, do not matter, because nobody remembers them. I asked dozens of cider vinegar fans about the theory behind it and none of them knew. Either they had never read Jarvis's books or they had forgotten the contents. People who sell the stuff don't know why they sell it. Maurice Hanssen has written a book on cider vinegar, but Jarvis's theory means nothing to him either. Here we have books which sold a million copies and founded an industry but the idea behind it all has vanished into oblivion. Only the cider vinegar remains, like the grin on the Cheshire Cat. And the joke is—it often works! People suffering from depression have picked up like magic after a few days on the stuff, but who knows why?

Q. *Why is yoghurt considered a wonder food?*
A. The large intestine has a resident population of bacteria, some "good", some "bad". The good ones, the acidophilus bacteria, synthesise B vitamins, so adding to the reserves. The bad bacteria putrefy food residues in the gut forming poisons which may be re-absorbed. Therefore anything which encourages the good bacteria and discourages the bad is an aid to health. Yoghurt, it is thought in some quarters, does this. The bacteria in it, either *lactobacillus bulgaricus* or *streptococcus thermophilus,* form lactic acid which in turn kills the putrefactive bacteria and feeds the friendly kind by supplying them with lactose. All this was discovered by Elie Metchnikoff, a Russian bacteriologist, early in this century. He noticed that the yoghurt-eating people of Bulgaria and Georgia tended to live longer than others and he propounded the theory that this was due to the control of putrefactive bacteria, and consequent reduction of poisons contributing to disease and senility.

Critics of the theory say that the souring bacteria in yoghurt are killed off by stomach acid long before they can reach the large intestine to do their good work. But not to worry. Yoghurt is still a good food. It contains protein, calcium and all the known vitamins.

Q. *Is there any proof that elixirs are beneficial?*
A. The common sense view of elixirs is that they contain vitamins and minerals in quantities too small to make a worthwhile contribution to diet, but possibly there are trace minerals which have some effect not yet discovered. Experiments in Switzerland with Biostrath have shown that it protects mice against the results of irradiation and that cancer patients undergoing ray treatment lose less weight and are generally less sick if they take Biostrath. It is not known why this is so.

Q. *What do tissue salts do?*
A. Most people taking them believe they are making good a deficiency, but this cannot possibly be so since the pills contain only one part per million of the salt. The treatment was introduced by Dr Schuessler during the last century. As Von Liebeg did with plants, he analysed the ash of human bodies to discover the mineral constituents. There were found to be twelve salts which he called biochemic tissue salts. These were then diluted and given in homoeopathic doses. The theory is that if you can by-pass the digestive tract, by absorbing the salt through the roof of the mouth, a tiny quantity is able to influence cell chemistry in some way which would be impossible through normal digestion. How it all works (if it does) is not really known. The process is different from homoeopathy, which is not really understood either. The main weakness of the system is the self-diagnosis required, involving a number of similar symptoms for different minor ailments, requiring different salts. A hypochondriac could have a field day without getting anywhere. But users insist that the benefits are there, and anyway the doses are harmless.

Q. *Why the growing enthusiasm for soya beans?*

A. Soya bean contains vegetable protein of high biological value. It has been called the miracle crop of the century. Soya fans point out that the beans are 40 per cent protein and weight for weight contain twice as much protein as meat, four times as much as eggs and twelve times as much as milk. All this assumes that you belong to the high protein school and want lots of it. Soya is particularly useful for vegetarians, who otherwise have a job knowing what to eat. Textured vegetable proteins, made of soya, are catching on but, says Dr Crawford (Chapter V), they lack EFA. Soya is also used as a source of plant milk for vegans, plant rennet for making vegetarian cheese, and lecithin.

Q. *How can a fertilised egg possibly be any different nutritionally from an unfertilised one?*
A. Whether it is fertilised or not cannot make any difference *per se.* But a fertilised egg is bound to be a free-range egg and in this case there is a difference, owing to the diet of the hen. According to Dr Crawford, a non-free-range egg contains twice as much saturated fat as a free-range egg.

Q. *What are so-called natural supplements derived from?*
A. Vitamins A and D—fish oils
        B   —brewers yeast, wheat germ, dried liver
        C and P—rose-hips, green peppers, orange juice and the latest discovery, acerola cherries. Some tablets are made of a mixture of these and some, if you don't watch out, have synthetic ascorbic acid added. Don't be conned by the advertising into thinking that acerola cherries, a very rich source, give you more for your money. A milligram is a milligram, whether from a rich source or a poor one.

E   —wheat germ oil
Lecithin—soya
Minerals—kelp (seaweed)

Q. *What are today's "wonder foods"?*
A. The same as yesterday's—yeast, wheat germ, yoghurt, molasses, honey, soya beans, liver—according to health food fans.

Yeast is recognised by all as a protein source containing all the B vitamins. It is thought that if the world continues galloping to destruction at the present rate, we shall have to grow yeast (which multiplies at a phenomenal rate) to keep going.

Wheat germ is a pleasant tasting source of all the B vitamins plus vitamin E and EFA. Can be eaten as a cereal by itself or added to granola. It is generally sold stabilised, which means that heat has been applied to destroy certain enzymes which hasten the breaking down of the nutrients.

Liver contains practically everything you need, because this is where all nutrients go en route from digestive tract to bloodstream and this is where many complex substances are built up. But being also the body's main filter, it may also contain some dubious items if the animal has had an artificial diet.

Yoghurt, molasses, soya and honey are dealt with above.

Q. *Has any explanation been put forward to account for inexplicable results claimed for certain foods?*
A. Results claimed for honey, pollen, ginseng, elixirs and possibly organic produce, cannot be explained in normal scientific terms. We fall back on that vague and unsatisfactory phrase "some mysterious X factor". It has been suggested that trace minerals, and possibly vitamins, may act synergistically so that each increases the effects of the others. So very small quantities, too small to be measured, might have quite

measurable results. There would be no X factor, just the adding up of minutiae which nobody thought worth considering or even knew about. But we shan't get the answer for awhile.

Q. *What about health farms? Don't they make a lot of money by just giving people nothing to eat?*
A. The popular idea of a health spa is that is where wealthy people go to reduce. But this is not the idea at all. According to the Nature Cure principles on which most health farms are run, you go to get rid of poisons. This is done by fasting, or going on a very reduced diet, so naturally you lose weight. But the weight loss is a bonus, not the sole object of the treatment.

Early in 1974, the *Daily Telegraph Magazine* ran a feature on health farms in which five guinea pigs had a week at different centres and the results were assessed in terms of cost for each pound of weight lost. General impressions were summarised by Dr Richard Gordon (author of *Doctor in the House).* He did not visit the centres himself and apparently made no attempt to find out the basis of the treatment, limiting his remarks to the slimming aspect. The verdict: "An expensive way of buying yoghurt."

A humorous writer naturally goes to town on the humorous side of the set-up—fat men on miniature bicycles, fat men being pinched and pummelled etc. He points out that massage does not reduce anybody but the masseuse, while ignoring its other objectives (stimulating circulation, toning up flabby muscles). Dr Gordon, in common with most people, finds the idea of an enema, "that weird speciality of health farms", fairly hilarious. Nobody told him (because he didn't ask) why they are given. If you accept the poison idea, the enema is logical. If you are getting rid of poisons you want them right out, not only half out. The large intestine only works normally when stimulated by solid foods; if you are fasting or living on juices it won't work, so the poisons which have come out from where they were lurking and got that far, must be helped over the final stage, otherwise the whole fast is a waste of time.

Like the general public, Dr Gordon is upset to think that you can pay $150 a week and upwards for the privilege of not eating. You could diet at home for free he thinks. But could you? Leaving out the little matter of willpower, you still have to pay rent, light and heat even if you don't eat. A three-star hotel would charge you the same price for a bed, without a single sip of carrot juice, or soothing words from the practitioner. No, the only people who can diet for nothing are tramps, and they don't need to.

The average health spa probably has as many staff as patients, when you count cleaners, gardeners and those who run the farm. This means that your fee equals the average wage plus rates, repairs, light, heat, consultants' fees, insurance and the cost of those few crumbs you get toward the end of your stay. Which doesn't leave so much for the wicked profiteer's fund.

Dr Gordon, still harping on dieting, is baffled about other motives. "It is impossible to say why customers, other than dieters, go to them" (health farms). Well, why do they? The vast majority vaguely want to "get fit". Unless they keep up the regimen—exercise and relaxation as well as diet—they are wasting their time. A few are hypochondriacs, a few go to relax from the stresses of the rat race, and push aside the sword of Damocles—a coronary—which always hangs over their heads. A minority are the last-ditchers, who have tried every cure in the medical world and still can't get well. Nature Cure is their last hope. Can it do anything for them? A lot depends on how late they have left it and how irreversible the condition is. Once the kidneys are damaged, you can't make new ones; once joints are deformed by arthritis, you can't put them straight. But you can halt most diseases and cure many more, say naturopaths. Provided the patient is willing to spend time, much can be done. Most people who go to a health farm are not prepared to spend time. Most expect to put right in two or three weeks the mistakes of several years. Time is always against the naturopath, for he has no fast-acting drugs to help him. If health farms continue to flourish, it must be because the word gets around.

CHAPTER IX

SUMMING UP

H AVING SUMMARIZED THE main ideas behind
food reform, what conclusions can we come to? Is it a lot of
hysterical nonsense (as official opinion has it) or has it a
logical basis? Perhaps a glance at food reformers themselves
might provide a clue.

There are three main groups, strange bedfellows at the best
of times, and if they occasionally agree it is due more to
chance than to any noticeable mental affinity. These groups
are (1) scientists, (2) commercial bandwagoners, and (3) those
who are usually lumped together by their opponents as emotional nitwits. This last group includes back-to-nature
enthusiasts, woolly-headed disciples of strange creeds,
hypochondriacs (who have read every health book there is)
and starry-eyed optimists, who feel that life ought to be better
than it is, and perhaps some magic formula exists to make it
so. Group 3, being for the most part without scientific
knowledge, tends to be at the mercy of Group 2, though it
would be unfair to suggest that all commercial people are
exploiters—some are idealists. If they make money by supplying a demand, that is no more than the rest of us do, from
archbishop to office cleaner.

It all comes back to human nature, which we discussed in
Chapter I. As long as there is a demand for the short-cut,
magic cure-all, somebody will supply it. Perhaps even a
scientist will supply it (though not commercially), as Metchnikoff did with yoghurt, or the Shutes with vitamin E. But on
the whole, scientist food reformers do not believe in wonder
foods or magic cures—they are more concerned with balance.

Balance is fast replacing the "have lots of" school of thought. You can have too much as well as too little of a good thing. Somebody has pointed out that even water in excess could be poison. And just as you can upset the balance by leaving something out, so you can upset it by putting too much of any one component in. Nothing illustrates the delicate balance—almost a knife-edge—between nutrients so well as the effect of protein in calcium absorption. Years ago, Dr Bircher-Benner of granola fame claimed that meat-eating led to bone porosity. Since he was a vegetarian and Nature Cure practitioner, this was regarded as the raving of a crank. But recent research indicates that calcium absorption is hindered by both too much and too little protein—you need to strike the happy medium.

The calcium-phosphorus team also includes vitamins D and B6 and magnesium. But once again there is a crucial balance. Too much magnesium, it is thought, also has an adverse effect on calcium absorption.

Then there is the cell-building team. We hear so often from protein propaganda that protein is the building and repair nutrient that we tend to overlook the other building materials—cholesterol, EFA and the phospholipids. Cholesterol is not a demon in itself, but only becomes so when its team partners are in short supply, inhibiting the building process, says Professor H. M. Sinclair. For the build-up of complex fatty acids from simple ones, vitamins E and B6 are needed. Fat is distributed by lecithin, a phospholipid which contains the B vitamins choline and inositol. Its action is speeded up by methionine, an amino acid. Lecithin can be made with the aid of an enzyme containing B6 and magnesium. So the cell-building team, which utilises cholesterol properly, consists of protein, EFA, several B vitamins, vitamin E and magnesium. If any of these ingredients are missing, cholesterol becomes no longer an asset but a liability.

We cannot possibly remember all these teams. It is enough to remember that team-work is the mainspring of the body's chemical activity, and any over-enthusiasm for one particular nutrient can throw the whole system out of gear. To ensure that all members of a team are present we need not to read books or swallow pills but to eat as varied a diet as possible.

When I was interviewing experts for this book, I met a nutritionist who said people should have better things to think about than what they eat. This seemed a strange creed for a nutritionist to hold, but one can see vaguely what he means. The idea is summed up more explicitly in a British Nutrition Foundation article. The author, Dr J. P. Greaves, points out that although knowledge of nutrient requirements plus knowledge of food composition might, in theory, enable one to work out a balanced diet, anyone who tried to do this in practice would end up a nervous wreck. "They would develop such a neurotic anxiety about their food that they would suffer in this way much more than they might possibly have done from any imbalance—imagined or otherwise—in their diets."

So if we want to keep out of the hypochondriac class of Group 3 among food reformers, we had better throw away our slide rules and give up trying to work out how many milligrams of vitamin C there are in a lettuce leaf, how many units of carotene in a carrot and how much calcium in a glass of milk. What we need is a bird's eye view of the whole business, not a detailed analysis.

This brings us to the big point on which food reformers are themselves divided—is the modern diet capable of providing all needed nutrients, or has it become so artificial that supplements (not necessarily pills) are advisable?

If we turn back to the research workers whose views are summarised in Chapter V (not all the authors were researchers) we find a strong conviction that artificial foods are the cause of most degenerative, or civilised, diseases, and that the solution lies not in taking supplements but in returning to a more natural diet. The main points are tabulated below.

None of these workers advocates the use of supplements. Mostly their diets are easily obtainable even in cities, though convenience foods, snacks, and restaurant meals would be out.

Researcher	Food denounced	Solution advised
Cleave	Refined carbohydrates	Cut out refined flour and sugar. Eat whole-wheat bread and fruits.
Yudkin	Refined sugar	Cut bought sugar to a minimum, get natural sugar from fruit.
Crawford	Processed foods and intensively reared animal foods which lack EFA	Whole grains, seeds, nuts, green vegetables, fish, more oil-containing fruits, meat of wild animals.
Bieler	Excess acid, stimulating and processed foods	Alkaline vegetables, unrefined foods, raw or undercooked protein in moderation.
Burkitt	Refined flour, denuded of fibre	Wholewheat bread, add bran to diet.
Various	Saturated fat	Cut saturated fat, increase PUFA.

Supporting these views we would find those food reformers who stress the value of whole foods. A whole food is, of course, an unrefined food. Its main attraction for the housewife is that it cuts out the need to calculate. If nothing has been taken out, and the diet is sufficiently varied, you can assume that all the team members are present. Its attraction for the worrier is the absence of additives.

If we now add the large body of opinion representing vegetarians and naturopathy, we find no quarrel with the

recommendations listed above, only an accent on the importance of fruit and vegetables as constituting more than half the
diet.

Where do health foods come in? Many health foods are
whole foods, but a great many are not, and there seems to be an
increasing tendency to jump on the convenience bandwagon.
So perhaps we can say that as long as you know what you
want, the health store may be a good place to get it, but if you
go just to look around, having read a confusing number of
health articles, you may end up with some very expensive nut
loaf and a basketful of bottles.

So let us suppose you are interested in food reform ideas,
without being either a scientist or salesman. Which section of
Group 3 do you fit into? Since most people would strongly
deny being eccentrics, let us assume you favour the back-to-
nature approach with the accent on whole foods. When your
friends ask what it's all about, you want to be able to give a
concrete explanation. Nothing hardens the cynic in his attitude
so much as equivocation, like the reply I got when I asked at a
food exhibition what was so great about pollen. "Well it's
natural isn't it, and natural things are better than artificial
things aren't they?" said the lady on the stand. When I pointed
out that Deadly Nightshade was natural she thought I was
wasting her time.

As we saw in Chapter IV a lot of silly stuff gets into the
organic farming propaganda which is a pity, since the idea
itself has a sound scientific basis. One supporter states: "Only
unchemicalised whole food is health-giving: chemicalised
vegetables are not only unhealthy but dangerous." Even if by
"chemicalised" the writer means sprayed, it is still nonsense
to suggest that spraying makes food any less whole. If he
means raised with artificial fertiliser, then he is even wider off
the mark, for fertiliser is not a poison—it would not be
required by the plant if it was. It is bad for the soil, may
perhaps inhibit the absorption of trace elements and by making
plants grow too fast it may lower their resistance to disease.
But to suggest that such plants poison the consumer only
weakens the case.

Whole foods come in for their share of propaganda too. A whole food, declares a supporter, is one "containing exactly the right balance of vitamins, minerals, starches and proteins, as nature provides". If a potato is exactly right, how can an orange, with much less starch, or a soya bean, with much more protein, also be exactly right? If every whole food is exactly right, why do we need a mixed diet at all?

There is a story which illustrates both man's need for variety and the folly of fanaticism. A fanatic decided that eggs were the perfect food, and since raw food is said to be better than cooked food he decided to eat his eggs raw. He died, because something in raw egg white knocks out biotin, a necessary B vitamin.

In addition to meaningless statements, the student of food reform needs to beware of myths. There are certain words which cannot pass the lips of the faddist without a shudder. These include cholesterol, saturated fat, starch and chemical.

Cholesterol, as we have seen, is essential to life. It is only under certain conditions of a badly balanced diet that it becomes dangerous.

Saturated fat, according to some writers, is "inert" and therefore useless. It clogs up the tissues, rather as grease clogs up the drain from the kitchen sink. This lurid picture is quite inaccurate. Saturated fat is an energy food, twice as effective in producing energy as carbohydrate or protein. Even when stored it does not clog up the tissues but remains available as a heat and energy supply for emergencies. (Very thin people are more likely to die of exposure.) It is only when saturated fat is eaten to excess, throwing the balance out, that trouble starts.

Starch is the word which makes dieters shudder. In excess it makes you fat, but you cannot live without it. In their efforts to cut starches, dieters tend to substitute high protein, but this may not be such a good idea either. Current theories suggest substituting vegetables and fruit.

The word chemical is anathema to lovers of the natural life. They forget that all plants, animals and humans are made up of chemicals, and plant nutrients in the soil are also chemicals, even in their natural state. Before bandying the word chemical around as a term of abuse, we should state clearly why a certain chemical is thought to be undesirable. Agricultural sprays, for instance, are designed to kill pests and are therefore poisonous in large quantities. Fertilisers, being plant foods, are not poisons as such, though they could be if taken in concentrated form. Chlorine dioxide, added to bread, is thought by some to destroy vitamin E and EFA; if this is so, then it is an objectionable chemical, but even this does not mean that all additives are poisons.

Some faddists believe that calcium is the stuff to take. (The official view is that we obtain our quota quite easily from a pint of milk a day plus the chalk in bread.) Rather than take a nasty chemical tablet, these people prefer to take dolomite (calcium and magnesium) which comes out of the ground. This, they think, is more "natural". But it doesn't include vitamins D and B6, vital members of the calcium team.

Balance means that the proportions in the diet as a whole (not each item) must be exactly right. Both food reformers and orthodox scientists agree on this. Where they disagree is on what the ideal proportions are and on the ability of the average diet to supply everything. Some favour high protein, some deny the importance of EFA, some say the fibre theory has not been proved, likewise the need for certain vitamins. So until the experts can agree, a whole-food diet seems the safest one to follow. If it supported primitive man for two million years, it should be good enough for us. It is the diet which all the arguments put forward in the table above point towards— whole grains and fruits for carbohydrate supply, meat from animals able to choose their food, more vegetables and fruit and more raw foods than the average modern diet contains. It's a simple solution, perhaps too simple for those who want us to live on ginseng and garlic tablets, or for those scientists who want to produce a polyunsaturated cow.

If a balanced diet leads to good health, it follows that rebalancing a faulty diet ought to bring a return to health if done in good time. This aspect of food reform has led to undue stress on cures and do-it-yourself medication. The enthusiast, having made a guess as to what deficiency might be at the root of his ill health, runs riot and takes excessive amounts of his wonder food, not realising that this excess will throw the balance out in the opposite direction. A sick person should consult an expert, either a doctor or a qualified naturopath, otherwise his guesswork may do more harm than good.

Do-it-yourself treatment is particularly dubious in the case of megavitamin therapy. It seems as though vitamins have a normal function which requires very small quantities, and possibly a therapeutic function in which very large doses are indicated. Not much is known about this latter aspect, so treatment is best left to an expert.

Normal re-balancing of the diet, without an excess of any one nutrient, should result in a gradual but permanent improvement in health, in contrast to the rapid action of the wonder drug with its side effects. But it is a comparatively slow process. Those in a hurry opt for the fast-acting drug or go berserk and take EFA by the quart, honey by the barrel or yeast by the sack. Those with patience may find that the tortoise wins in the end. This is shown most dramatically in the case of arthritis, which orthodox medicine insists is incurable. Innumerable cases have in fact been cured by diet, but expert advice is still essential in all cases of major illness.

If the first aim of a diet is to keep fit and the second to cure something, the third and most ambitious aim is to prolong life. There are three aspects of diet said to prevent ageing:

1. Taking sufficient Vitamin E to prevent the oxidation of EFA which leads to cell breakdown.
2. Reducing protein intake after middle age.
3. Eating very little altogether.

All these theories have been proved with animals. Are there any humans around to uphold them? If we look at existing healthy, long-lived communities, we find they all have certain things in common. The best known examples are the Hunzas (mentioned in Chapter IV), the people of Georgia and Azerbaijan in the Caucasus, and a newly discovered community in the Vilcabamba valley of Ecuador. What they have in common is that all eat an unrefined, mainly vegetarian diet (with a little meat), all eat sparingly and all are mountain people.

Hunza has been called the land of just enough. Having no sophisticated storage methods, the people go hungry in spring when supplies run low and new crops have not yet come up. In Vilcabamba, the average daily intake is said to be 1,700 calories, which would be a strict reducing diet in an affluent country. In addition to their sparse meals, all these communities are physically active, tilling the land on steep hillsides. The Georgians are so energetic that their orchestra of centenarians not only plays merry tunes, but they dance to them at the same time, an accomplishment which exhausts the audience more than the performers.

This all links up with the theory, held by many, that exercise is every bit as important to health as diet. Professor Yudkin in his anti-sugar book, remarks jokingly that the incidence of coronary heart disease correlates with the number of TV sets just as closely as it does with diet. I would make a guess that it also correlates inversely with dog licences (anybody with a dog has to do *some* walking). Many food reformers blame the rise in degenerative diseases on the increase in food refining this century. But is food refining the only major change in our lives? The coming of the internal combustion engine seems equally important, closely followed by the advent of television. One gets us home from work quickly and the other keeps us there. Against such unnatural conditions, even the best diets may fail to maintain health.

Dr K. H. Cooper, author of *Aerobics* (an exercise system), claims that the blood cholesterol of a fit person returns to normal after a fatty meal in less than half the time taken by an unfit person. Exercise also does these things for you: it increases the effectiveness of lungs and heart, increases the number and size of blood vessels, improves muscle tone and elasticity of arteries, helps elimination of poisons by increased sweating, releases tension, and last but not least, ''can change your whole outlook on life. You learn to relax, sleep better and get more work done with less fatigue''. Anyone for jogging?

Unfortunately, affluence and lack of exercise go together. What do the well-to-do spend money on? Nine times out of ten on houses, furniture, labour-saving devices, vehicles, hi-fi equipment, food, drink and entertainment—all part of the sedentary life. Few millionaires buy squash racquets or climbing boots—if they did, they would be hard pressed to find an outlet for their money.

Then there is a final factor which, while not a food, is interwoven with diet and exercise in determining our final state of health. This is worry or stress.

Worry is an offshoot of fear, and fear, we may remember, stimulates the primitive endocrine system (which we still have) to prepare for fight or flight. If no physical action follows the alarms, the chemical reactions have taken place for nothing and all sorts of side effects may result, as we saw when considering atherosclerosis. In addition to increasing the risk of heart disease, stress is said to: raise blood pressure, impair absorption and utilisation of food, cause breakdown of cell protoplasm, use up potassium (hence arthritis), vitamins B and C and lecithin, waste energy, and by causing muscle tension during sleep, produce excess lactic acid which irritates nerves. So in addition to worrying about poisons, deficiencies and pollution, the worriers now have to worry about worry.

But all is not lost says Gayelord Hauser. If you make sure of all the calcium team from food sources (not rock) you can say goodbye to the worry habit. People suffering from ''exhaustion, nervousness, excitability, irritability, apprehension and insomnia'' recovered dramatically, he claims, when given sufficient B6 (lost during flour refining) along with the rest of the team. Since 90 per cent of the population suffer from at least some of the above symptoms, the tendency to try a new pill is immense. But if the manufacturer is not team-minded, something may be missing from the pill. The only reliable pill, it seems, is whole food, which supplies all the ingredients without your having to think.

Can we therefore say that a whole-food diet can supply all
our needs? Provided it is balanced and varied, the answer
should be yes. We ought to be able to get everything with knife
and fork. If we don't it is because the lure of the ready-made
dish is too strong, because we don't like greens, or prefer pies
to fresh fruit. It is estimated by pessimists that in the average
diet, two-thirds of the calories are supplied by devitalised
foods.

However, most foods are obtainable in whole form, i.e.:

Carbohydrates	Wholewheat bread, potatoes, root vegetables
Proteins	Eggs (preferably free-range), fresh fish, milk (preferably unpasteurised), nuts, peas, and beans
Vitamins and minerals	Fresh fruits, vegetables

Needless to say all these foods, being whole foods, are mixtures of nutrients—there is protein in bread, carbohydrate in
milk and vitamins and minerals distributed throughout all.
Meat is not included as a whole food because it can no longer
be described as a food with nothing added, nothing taken
away. As we have seen, meat produced under intensive farming conditions has an unnaturally high ratio of saturated to
unsaturated fat. Unless you move in grouse-shooting, stag-
hunting circles you are unlikely to get meat which has not been
artificially raised. Perhaps mutton from hill sheep is the near-
est approach, though not all sheep are left to look after themselves. But there is still plenty of fresh fish around. (However,
watch out for mercury.)

The big advantage of a varied natural diet, according to
nutritionists, is that there is an unexpected bonus. Not only do
you get all the ingredients, but they react on each other so that

the combined effect is greater than that of the sum of the parts.

If the simple expedient of a varied whole-food diet is the answer to all our problems, why is there so much argument on the subject of nutrition? Why are there so many fad diets, why do extremists take twenty or more pills a day, and why is orthodox opinion so violently opposed to any criticism of food processing?

If we track all these items to their source we come to the crux of the situation—population explosion. Because population has increased, there has been a mass migration to towns with consequent food transport problems, and there has been a vastly increased demand for food. By means of modern technology, these problems have been solved. A varied diet is available for the town dweller. Everything is hygienic, nothing goes bad. A hundred years ago, given towns of the present size, this would have been impossible—either food poisoning would have been the order of the day, or supplies would have been inadequate.

But this great achievement has made us arrogant, and in our blind faith in science we have made mistakes which are only just beginning to come to light. Some people are still denying that they are mistakes. But according to food reformers, they are:

1. Refining, which alters the balance of the nutrients. Though losses occur, these can perhaps be made good from other sources. The most serious effect of refining seems to be the unnatural concentration of what remains.

2. In an effort to supply increasing demand, technology has speeded up natural processes. Both crops and animals are made to grow faster, eggs are laid more frequently. In the case of animals, this has altered the balance of fats, because there is less time to build up the long-chain PUFAs. In the case of crops, EFA is also reduced and there is greater susceptibility to disease, necessitating sprays which add to cost and cause pollution.

3. In an effort to counteract some of the problems now appearing, technology concentrates on cure rather than prevention. Sugar causes tooth decay, so we put fluorine in the water instead of going easy on soft drinks. (Some say fluorine inhibits enzyme activity, without which we cannot live.) In a frantic effort to control the heart disease explosion, scientists are trying to artificially manipulate the composition of cow's milk instead of concentrating on the source of the trouble. And at the back of every technological mind is the thought that if all else fails, potent wonder drugs are at hand to deal with our ailments, and even transplants may be the answer.

These failings are not on the whole admitted by orthodox nutritionists. Since they know more about the dangers of contamination than we do, they attach more importance to hygiene than to wholeness. Refining certainly makes for hygiene—there is no unstable element left to go bad. But with modern storage, packaging and refrigeration it is no longer essential; it remains because we have got used to the attractive appearance of refined foods. Preservatives help further by keeping bacteria at bay. We could hardly be safer in the short term. And because technologists are not prophets the long-term snags were not foreseen. Now that some awkward people are pointing them out, there is controversy. Those responsible for our nice hygienic world do not like to think there is anything wrong with it. And who can blame them? Similarly, those who have found a way to give us more food faster, do not like to think there is anything wrong with the food they produce. So we can expect the status quo to be defended strongly for some time to come.

On the other side of the fence we have the worriers, who are susceptible to propaganda of all kinds, scientific and otherwise. Since food reformers tend to go in for detail (somebody has written a whole book, just on magnesium) the public gets its information in dribs and drabs, like the mouse who saw an elephant's toe one day, its tail another and its trunk after that. The mouse had no idea what the elephant really looked like— and the worrier has not much idea what goes on either; he only knows he is worried about poisons and deficiencies, hence the taking of innumerable supplements and the experimenting with strange diets.

At the beginning of this chapter we asked, "Is food reform a lot of hysterical nonsense?" The answer seems to be—some of it is and some of it isn't. Perhaps this review of current ideas may help us to discern a pattern, so that eventually we can decide what the elephant looks like, despite the jungle which surrounds him.

DIALOGUE

Q. *Talking about balance, is the acid/alkali balance of the diet generally thought to be important?*
A. What is meant by acid and alkali? For a simple scientific explanation you can't do better than read the relevant sections of *The A to Z of Health Food Terms* contributed by Dr R. F. Milton. As for the balance in the diet, it is thought by some to be vital, by others of no importance. Here are some opinions:

"This is another happy hunting ground of the faddist . . . it is unimportant if kidneys are healthy" *(Food and Principles of Dietetics);* "Proteins maintain the balance by combining with whichever is in excess" (Hauser); "The natural buffering of the blood takes care of it automatically" (doctor); "You need something to buffer with, i.e. adequate alkaline-forming foods in the diet" (Naturopath); "Excess acid makes for tired and cramped muscles, increasing with age" (health writer); "Forget it" (Nutrition teacher); "Some eminent physicians now believe that the diseases of the blood vessels which are responsible for high blood pressure, kidney disease, gangrene and apoplexy are the results of prolonged injury due to eating excessive amounts of acid-forming foods'' (Dr E. V. McCollum, Johns Hopkins University); ''Without this acid-base balance, good health is impossible to maintain'' (Dr H. G. Bieler, author of *Food Is Your Best Medicine).*

Even if you don't want to forget it, you can't be perpetually consulting tables when eating, so perhaps a good general rule may be just to increase the amount of fruit and vegetables in your diet. These are for the most part alkaline in reaction, provided you don't add sugar to fruit or overcook vegetables. Fresh fruits and raw vegetables 'have many benefits and most of us don't eat nearly enough of them.

Q. *How do special diets fit into the whole-food scheme?*
A. Mostly they don't. The Hay Diet, popular in the 1930s but now almost forgotten, was based on the theory that since different nutrients such as starch and protein are acted on by different digestive juices, taking them at the same meal would cause havoc in the digestive tract. So you had to have your poached egg without toast. The idea comes unstuck when you realise that natural foods are mixtures of nutrients though one may predominate, like starch in bread. Some people, with very delicate digestions, seem to benefit by avoiding too much mixing, but the average person doesn't need to bother.

The juice cure has a number of followers. Juices provide a quick and easy way to get vitamins and minerals from fruits and vegetables. People who do not like vegetables, and therefore are likely to be deficient, find it easier to drink the juice. But juice is very concentrated and lacking in fibre. Any liquid diet could be dangerous without an enema (see under Health Farms, Chapter VIII), because toxic wastes would accumulate and possibly damage the kidneys. Naturopaths recommend diluted juices during a supervised fast, but not as a regular thing.

The grape cure, which excited a lot of interest by claiming to cure cancer, is what is known as a mono-diet, meaning a diet of one ingredient only. It is thought that by reducing digestive activity to a minimum, an exhausted system has a chance to recover. But this is the very reverse of a balanced diet and not intended for normal people.

Then there are some fancy reducing diets such as steak and pineapple, milk and bananas etc. If they succeed, it is probably because the very monotony reduces intake. The high fat reducing diet is condemned by all except its supporters as being dangerous. The advantage of the rice diet is supposed to be its lack of salt. But extreme salt restriction should be supervised by a doctor. All these diets are unbalanced.

Q. *What is so special about fresh raw food? Why do health farms and fancy clinics recommend it?*
A. We have to distinguish between fresh food and raw food— they are not always the same. As we saw in Chapter VI, you can eat salads which are far from fresh. You can eat nuts left over from last Christmas or apples stored for months, but they are not fresh either. All the ''miracle cures'' related by Nature Cure enthusiasts relate to fresh or live foods which have had no time to deteriorate. Even meat, when freshly killed, contains some vitamin C which will very soon disappear. As soon as a food is harvested, cellular change begins and enzymes start to break down. (Although we have our own digestive enzymes, those in fresh foods help.) Does freshness only involve enzymes and unstable vitamins, or is there a magic something not yet identified? Swedish scientists think there is, and have named the mystery factor auxones. Nobody knows much about them but there is a claim that they increase the micro-electric tension in the cell, with beneficial results. This whole business of micro-electric tension is a new field that we shall be hearing more about in future (see Chapter IV).

Raw food, to be at its best, should come out of your own garden or straight off the farm where it grew. Perhaps labour costs are a blessing in disguise if they result in more ''pick your own fruit'' signs outside farms. But even if you live in a high-rise apartment, there is still hope. We are told that the most "live" food you can have is sprouted seeds, and the sprouting can be done at home. During sprouting, the vitamin content soars; the nutrients in sprouting seeds are building up, not breaking down. A health food store should be able to supply suitable seeds and instructions on how to do the sprouting.

Q. *What are the main snags in present-day food and eating habits from the food reform angle?*
A. The snags, say food reformers, are in the eating habits rather than the foods themselves. Good food can be obtained if you know what to pick. With three-quarters of the population living in towns, most of whom go out to work, the order of the day is: breakfast (packaged cereal with tea or coffee, bolted down at top speed) and a midday meal out. If this meal is taken in a restaurant, it will be for the most part over-cooked and warmed up. Since labour is now more costly than ingredients, canned vegetables predominate, and you just can't avoid French fries. Canned fruit may be the alternative to a stodgy pudding or pie, which the caterers think men must have. At the other end of the scale from the bought meal is the lunchbox of sandwiches. There is no reason why a packed lunch should not be first rate nutrition, but it rarely is. In between, we get the snack-bar lunchers, who are either dieting or economising (though in fact they achieve neither). Coffee and a bun may give a sense of virtue, but it gives little nourishment.

The packed lunch people have their main meal in the evening, usually in competition with the TV. The others have a snack on a tray. In both cases there is a tendency for the meal to consist of convenience foods, so that the person preparing it can get back to the TV as fast as possible. Those who for some reason have missed out, fill up with biscuits, coffee and bottled drinks. Meals like this will consist of:

1. Excess sugar (in biscuits, cakes, canned fruit, ice cream, bottled drinks).

2. Excess starch (in biscuits, cakes, sandwiches, rolls, pies, potatoes, puddings).
3. Badly cooked vegetables, insufficient fresh vegetables, fresh fruit and salads.
4. Excess saturated fat (in fried snacks, fried fish, pastry, puddings, biscuits and ice cream).
5. Possible shortage of water-soluble vitamins and minerals unless made up at home.
6. Shortage of EFA and vitamin E due to predominance of processed foods.
7. Excess stimulants (tea, coffee and cola drinks throughout the day).

The authorities would agree with most of this. They deplore excess starch, sugar, fat and bad cooking, but like to believe, with obstinate optimism, that these things are the exception. The point official opinion might not agree on is No 6, shortage of EFA. While PUFAs are accepted as a possible cure for high cholesterol, few people are particularly interested in their role in normal nutrition. Those who are concerned about it feel that this neglect is serious. (See Chapter V.)

BIBLIOGRAPHY

Adams, Ruth, and Frank Murray. *Megavitamin Therapy.* New York: Pinnacle Books, 1975.

Arnow, E. Earle. *Food Power: A Doctor's Guide to Common-sense Nutrition.* Chicago: Nelson-Hall Co., 1972.

Atkins, Robert C. *Dr. Atkins' Diet Revolution: The High Calorie Way to Stay Thin Forever.* New York: David McKay Co., Inc., 1972.

Bieler, H. G. *Food Is Your Best Medicine.* New York: Random House, 1966.

Bircher-Benner Clinic. *Bircher-Benner Raw Food and Juices Nutrition Plan.* New York: Nash Publishing Corp., 1972.

Chase, Alice. *Nutrition for Health.* Englewood Cliffs, N.J.: Prentice-Hall, 1967.

Davis, Adelle. *Let's Eat Right to Keep Fit.* New York: Harcourt Brace Jovanovich, 1970.

Dickie, R. S. *Diet in Health and Disease.* Springfield, Ill.: Charles C. Thomas, Publishers, 1975.

DiCyan, Erwin. *The Truth About Vitamin E.* New York: Bantam Books, 1973.

———. *The Vitamins in Your Life.* New York: Simon & Schuster, Inc., 1975.

Dietary Allowances and Committee & Food & Nutrition Board. *Recommended Dietary Allowances, 8th Edition.* Washington, D.C.: National Academy of Sciences, 1974.

Ebon, Martin. *Which Vitamins Do You Need?.* New York: Bantam Books, 1974.

Evans, E. V. *The World of Food and Nutrition.* New York: Panther House, Ltd., 1971.

Fisher, Patty, and Arnold E. Bender. *The Value of Food*. New York: Oxford University Press, 1975.

Fredericks, Carlton. *The Nutrition Handbook: Your Key to Good Health*. Chatsworth, Cal.: Major Books, 1975.

Fredericks, Carlton, and Herbert Bailey. *Food Facts and Fallacies*. New York: Arc Books, 1968.

Fried, John J. *The Vitamin Conspiracy*. New York: Saturday Review Press, 1975.

Grant, Doris. *Recipe for Survival: Your Daily Food*. New Canaan, Conn.: Keats Publishing, Inc.

Hall, Ross. *Food for Nought: The Decline of Nutrition*. New York: Harper & Row Publishers, Inc., 1974.

Hauser, Gayelord. *Look Younger, Live Longer*. New York: Farrar, Straus & Giroux, Inc., 1951.

Hunter, Beatrice T. *Natural Foods Primer*. New York: Simon and Schuster, Inc., 1973.

Hunter, Kathleen. *Health Foods and Herbs*. New York: Arc Books, 1968.

Kordel, Lelord. *Eat and Grow Younger*. New York: Manor Books, 1973.

———. *Health Through Nutrition*. New York: Manor Books, 1973.

Kotschevar, L. H., and Margaret McWilliams. *Understanding Foods*. New York: John Wiley & Sons, Inc., 1969.

Lappe, Frances M. *Diet for a Small Planet*. New York: Ballantine Books, 1975.

Latour, John. *The ABC's of Vitamins, Minerals and Natural Foods*. New York: Arc Books, 1972.

Leverton, Ruth M. *Food Becomes You: Better Health Through Better Nutrition*. New York: Doubleday & Co., Inc., 1965.

McWilliams, Margaret. *Food Fundamentals, 2nd Edition*. New York: John Wiley & Sons, Inc., 1974.

Marsh, Edward E. *How to Be Healthy with Natural Foods*. New York: Arco Publishing Co., Inc., 1967.

Miller, Marjorie. *Introduction to Health Foods*. Plainview, N.Y.: Nash Publishing Corporation, 1971.

Morton, H. A. *Fat Soluble Vitamins*. Elmsford, N.Y.. Pergamon Press, Inc., 1970.

Null, Gary, and Steve Null. *The Complete Handbook of Nutrition*. New York: Dell Publishing Company, 1973.

Passwater, Richard. *Supernutrition: The Megavitamin Revolution*. New York: The Dial Press, 1975.

Pauling, Linus. *Vitamin C and the Common Cold*. San Francisco: W. H. Freeman and Company, 1970.

Pritzker, Wendy. *Natural Foods and Vitamins Handbook*. New York: Arc Books, 1974.

Pyke, Magnus. *Man and Food*. New York: McGraw-Hill, 1970.

Robinson, Corrine. *Basic Nutrition and Diet Therapy, 3rd Edition*. New York: Macmillan, Inc., 1975.

Rodale, J. I. *The Complete Book of Vitamins*. Emmaus, Pa.: Rodale Press.

———. *The Complete Book of Food and Nutrition*. Emmaus, Pa.: Rodale Press.

Shute, Wilfred E. *Dr. Wilfred E. Shute's Complete, Updated Vitamin E Book*. New Canaan, Conn.. Keats Publishing Inc., 1975.

Tatkon, D. *The Great Vitamin Hoax*. New York: Macmillan, 1967.

Turner, Dorothea. *Handbook of Diet Therapy*. Chicago: University of Chicago Press, 1970.

Wade, Carlson. *Fact-Book on Vitamins and Other Food Supplements*. New Canaan, Conn.: Keats Publishing Company, Inc., 1972.

Winter, Ruth. *Vitamin E: The Miracle Worker*. New York: Arc Books, 1972.

Yudkin, J. *Sweet and Dangerous*. New York: Bantam Books, 1973.

INDEX

Acid, 40, 48, 51, 54, 68, 90, 114, 115, 116, 127, 135, 142, 152, 161, 171–2

Acrolein, 137

Additives, 13, 16, 113, 120–24, 129–30, 142, 149, 161, 164

Adrenals, adrenalin, 24, 28, 80, 100, 118, 127–8

Agene, 122, 129

Ageing, 122, 129

Alcohol, 28, 29

Alkaline, 12, 34, 40, 48, 51, 54, 90, 91, 115, 116, 127, 131, 136, 142, 161, 171–2

Allinson, Dr. T.R., 108

American Nutrition Foundation, 47

Amino acid, 23, 27, 30, 31, 110

Anemia, 24, 105, 110, 115

Antibiotic, 16, 39, 63, 96, 107, 111, 122–23, 142

Anti-oxidant, 89–90, 95, 112, 113

Arachidonic acid, 114

Artery: arteries; damage; disease; arteriosclerosis; atheroma; atherosclerosis, 49, 74, 75, 76, 81, 82–84, 132, 135, 166

Bacteria, 25, 43, 47, 57–60, 124, 134, 152, 170

Balfour, Lady Eve, 57, 62

Benzoic acid, 97

Beri-beri, 88, 93

Bieler, Dr. H.G., 65, 77, 126–28, 135–36, 161

Bile, 25, 34, 126, 135

Bioflavanoids, 112

Biological value (protein), 27, 31–32, 50

Biotin, 107, 110, 163

Bircher-Benner, Dr., 38–39, 44, 159

Blood pressure, 74, 84, 114, 133, 134, 167

Blood vessels, 25, 33, 80, 113, 134, 166

Botulism, 123

Bran, 66, 94, 109–10, 142, 144, 161
Bread, 23, 52, 77, 79, 93, 94, 107–9, 129–33, 138, 142–44, 150, 161
Breast feeding, 83, 95
Burkitt, D.P., 65, 78–79, 161

Caffeine, 28, 29, 100, 134
Calcium, 24, 25, 49, 78, 88, 89, 90, 93, 102, 109, 112, 115–17, 125, 133, 144, 152, 153, 159, 164, 167
Calorie, 23, 31
Cancer, 64, 72, 79, 123, 135, 173
Carbohydrate (see also Starch), 22–23, 26, 27, 29–30, 41, 52, 53, 65–71, 81, 88, 92–93, 116, 131, 134, 161, 163, 164, 168
Carbon, 20, 23, 32
Carbon dioxide, 22, 26
Carotene, 89, 143, 160
Chiropractice, 48
Chlorinated water, 77, 78, 100, 124
Chlorine, 78, 90
Chlorine dioxide, 100, 122, 129, 132, 164
Cholesterol, 29, 33, 45, 67, 72–79, 81–84, 96, 106, 111–12, 118, 131, 132, 144, 159, 163, 166, 175

Choline, 81, 159
Cider vinegar, 144, 151–52
Cleave, T.L., 65, 78, 161
Cobalt, 119
Co-enzyme, 25, 103
Collagen, 25, 88, 96, 112
Comfrey, 43
Compost, 56, 57–61
Copper, 119
Coronary: heart disease (CHD); thrombosis, 18, 27, 28, 42, 45, 64, 65, 67, 70–79, 80–83, 84–85, 90, 112, 113, 138, 151, 166, 167, 170
Cortisone, 118
Crawford, Dr. M.A., 65, 75–77, 114, 154
Cyclamates, 122

Davis, Adelle, 45–46, 47, 83, 115, 117, 136, 145
DDT, 120–21, 128–29
Deficiency, 11, 12, 15, 17–18, 26–27, 45, 49, 128, 143–44, 153, 167, 171, 172
Degenerative diseases, 18, 64–85, 160, 166
Dental decay; cavities, 68, 70, 72, 124–25, 131, 170
Diabetes, 66–70, 72, 132, 138, 151
Digestion, 25, 30
Diseases of civilization (see Degenerative diseases)

Diverticular disease, 68, 79, 80, 132
Dolomite, 164

Ecology, 51, 56, 121, 139
EFA (*see* Fatty acid)
Elimination, 26, 38, 44, 49, 125–6, 127, 135
Elixers, 144–46, 153, 155
Endocrine glands, 24, 113–14, 127, 167
Energy, 19, 22–23, 26–30, 93, 115, 117, 125, 131–32, 167
Enzymes, 24–26, 60, 87, 93, 95, 113, 116, 117, 125, 128, 144, 155, 159, 170, 173
Eskimos, 27, 30, 51, 53, 56, 74, 77, 136
Essential amino acids, 27, 31
Essential fatty acids (*see* Fatty acid)
Evolution, 51–54, 65, 69, 70
Excretion, 26, 49
Exercise, 11, 18, 49, 61, 74, 82, 85, 166–67

Fasting, 37, 40, 127, 156, 157, 172
Fat, 22–23, 25, 27–28, 29, 30, 32, 67–68, 71, 72, 73, 74, 75, 76, 78, 81, 82, 84–85, 88, 90, 99, 100, 120, 131, 134–35, 173

Fat, animal: saturated, 28, 32, 42, 45, 54, 67–68, 70, 73, 74, 75, 81, 84–85, 134–35, 137, 147, 154, 161, 163, 168, 175
structural: unsaturated, 27–28, 30, 33, 54, 75–77, 84–85, 95, 134–35, 168
Fatty acid:
essential (EFA), 28, 32–33, 75–77, 81, 83, 107, 112–14, 117, 123, 124, 129, 132–43, 147, 155, 159, 161, 164, 165, 170, 175
polyunsaturated (PUFA), 32–33, 81, 83, 85, 94, 135, 161, 164, 170, 175
Fiber, 68, 78–79, 80–81, 92, 94, 108, 132, 134, 144, 161, 164, 172
Flour, 27, 52, 92, 107–10, 142, 150, 161
Fluorine, 102, 124, 130, 134, 170
Food and Drug Administration, 13, 47, 127

Gastric acid, 69, 116
Georgia (old people of), 151, 152, 165–66
Ginseng, 149–50, 164
Glucose (blood sugar), 23, 28–30, 66, 82, 100, 106, 128, 134, 148

Glucose (commercial), 148
Glycogen, 30, 66, 117
Graham, Sylvester, 108
Grape cure, 44, 173

Hauser, Gayelord, 11, 15, 36, 43–46, 145, 171
Hay diet, 172
Health food, 47, 78, 91, 128, 138–57, 161
Health food stores, 14, 37, 39, 45, 92, 94, 128, 162, 174
Health spas, 47, 48, 156–57, 173
Heart: attack; disease (*see* Coronary)
Honey, 143–44, 148, 151, 155, 165
Hormones, 16, 24, 28, 72, 90, 113, 123–24, 131, 142
Hunzas, 55–56, 165–66
Hydrogen, 23, 32
Hydrogenation, 32, 45
Hypoglycemia, 66

Indigestion, 72
Inglis, Brian, 39
Inositol, 81–82, 159
Insecticide (*see* Pesticide)
Insulin, 66, 72
Intensive farming, 17, 46, 54, 71, 76, 84–85, 142, 168
Iodine, 24
Iron, 24, 90, 92, 100, 109, 110, 115, 116, 144

Kelp, 143–44, 150, 155
Ketone, 30
Kidneys, 23, 26, 29, 40, 49, 127
Kordel, Lelord, 15, 45–46, 50, 145

La Leche League, 95
Laxative, 19
Lecithin, 45, 81–82, 117, 144, 154, 159, 167
Lief, Stanley, 14, 39
Linoleic acid, 75, 77, 114
Linolenic acid, 114
Liver, 25, 30, 34–35, 43, 80–83, 126–27
Liver salts, 12, 34, 49
Lungs, 22, 26, 40, 127, 166

McCance, R.A., 108–9
McCarrison, Sir Robert, 47, 54–56, 61, 63, 80, 109
Macrobiotics, 47, 48
Magnesium, 82, 90, 101, 117, 144, 159, 164, 170
Margarine, 28, 32, 35, 74, 77, 89, 143
Masai, 71, 74, 77, 82, 136
Meat, 40–46, 48, 50, 135–36, 142, 154, 159, 161, 164, 168, 173
Megavitamin, 165
Mental health, 34, 64, 79–80
Metabolism, 22–29, 30, 37, 40, 49, 88, 93, 103, 106, 116, 131, 134

Metchnikoff, Elie, 152, 158
Methionine, 159
Milk, 23, 42, 53, 89, 95, 102, 116, 135, 142, 154, 164, 168, 170
Minerals, 12, 22–24, 40, 66, 80, 86–87, 90–92, 95, 98, 102, 104, 107, 111, 114–18, 132, 144–48, 150, 153, 155, 163, 168, 172, 174
Molasses, 44, 150–51, 155

Nature Cure, 15, 16, 37–41, 43, 44, 45, 47, 108, 110, 126, 138, 145, 156, 157, 159, 165, 173
Naturopath; Naturopathy, 11, 35, 39, 45, 46, 47, 48, 68, 78, 125, 157, 161, 171, 172
Niacin, 24, 88, 93, 103, 104, 107, 110
Nitrates; Nitrites; Nitrosamines, 123
Nitrogen, 23, 26, 31, 49, 58, 135

Obesity, 66, 72, 85, 131, 138
Oil, 28, 32, 76, 77, 83, 89, 92, 94–95, 99, 105, 110, 112, 114, 134–35, 143, 147, 148, 155, 161
Organic farming; organic produce, 14, 47, 57, 63, 139, 141, 142, 144, 145, 146, 156, 162

Osmosis, 72–73, 97
Osteopathy, 48
Osteoporosis, 49, 159
Oxalic acid, 102, 116
Oxidation, 22–23, 27–28, 129
Oxygen, 22–23, 25, 34

Painter, N., 65, 78
Pancreas, 24, 113
Pantothenic acid, 106, 110
Pasteurization, 95, 97, 102, 116, 135–36, 148, 150, 168
Patent medicines, 12, 72, 141
Pauling, Dr. Linus, 47, 96–97
Pellagra, 88, 104
Pesticide, 16, 57, 113, 120–21, 128–29, 130
Phospholipid, 81, 159
Phosphorus, 24–25, 58, 88, 90, 108, 111, 116, 159
Phosphotase, 116
Phytic acid, 116
Pituitary, 24, 127
Poison (toxin); Poisoning (see also Toxaemia), 11–14, 16–17, 19, 25, 29–30, 34, 37–38, 39–42, 44, 47, 49, 63, 96, 113, 120–37, 142, 145, 152, 156, 157, 162, 164, 166, 172, 180
Pollen, 149, 156, 162
Polyunsaturated fatty acid (PUFA) (see Fatty acid)

Potassium, 24, 58, 90, 101, 118, 144, 150–51, 167

Preservatives, 13, 16, 29, 97, 123, 132, 149, 170

Price, Dr. J.A., 78, 123, 124, 132

Primitive diet; Primitive man, 51–54, 61, 76, 84, 97, 136, 139, 164

Processing, 12, 29, 62, 123, 129–30, 134, 149, 150, 161, 169–70

Protein, 22–23, 24, 27, 30–31, 37, 41–43, 45–46, 49–50, 52, 63, 65, 69, 76, 92, 106, 108, 116, 127, 132, 135–36, 142, 152–55, 159, 168, 172

PUFA (see Fatty acid)

Purine, 134, 135

Pyridoxine (B6), 82, 103, 106, 110, 116, 117, 159, 164, 167

Pyruvic acid, 27, 93, 116

Refining, 16, 17, 26, 40, 44, 46, 53, 54, 62–63, 67, 68, 69, 70, 71, 73, 76, 77, 80, 82, 86, 90, 102, 115, 121, 132, 161, 167, 170

Rheumatism, 49, 62, 112, 134

Riboflavin (B2), 49, 93, 95, 101, 103

Rice, 27, 67, 69, 88, 92, 130, 133

Rickets, 61, 88–89, 116–17

Rodale, J.I., 15, 65, 79, 145

Saccharine disease, 65–70, 71, 73, 78, 79, 131–32

Salt (table), 17, 97, 117, 127, 130, 133, 141, 143, 148, 173

Saturated fat (see Fat)

Scurvy, 88, 96, 111, 112

Shute, Dr. E., 90, 94, 158

Sinclair, Hugh, 75, 159

Skin, 26, 38, 40, 49

Sodium, 24, 90, 102, 117–18, 147

Soya bean, 153–54, 155

Sprouting, 174

Stanton, Dr. G., 65, 78, 81, 123, 124, 132

Starch (see also Carbohydrate), 23, 37, 50, 77, 78, 127, 163, 174, 175

Stefansson, 27, 133, 136

Stimulants, 28–29, 49, 82, 100, 127–28, 134, 136, 161, 175

Stress, 11, 18, 29, 50, 74, 80–82, 100, 157, 166–67

Sugar, blood (see Glucose)

Sugar, white, refined, 17, 23, 27, 49, 50, 65–77, 79, 80, 84, 92, 93, 102, 107, 131–33, 138, 140, 143, 147, 149, 151, 161, 170, 172, 174–75

Sulphur, 90

Sulphur dioxide, 97, 99, 142, 147
Supplements, 12, 19, 90, 105–6, 143–44, 149, 154, 160, 171
Sweat, 26, 40, 167

Tension, 28, 80, 82, 167
Tissue salts, 140–41, 144, 153
Thiamine (B₁), 49, 88, 97, 99, 103, 106, 110
Thyroid, 24
Tooth decay (see Dental decay)
Toxaemia, 126–27, 136
Trace elements (trace minerals), 17, 24, 59, 90, 130, 144, 146, 150, 153, 155, 162
Triglyceride (see Fat)
Tryptophan, 24–25, 109

Ulcer, 64, 69, 73, 132
Unsaturated fat (see Fat)
Urea, 49
Uric acid, 49, 81, 118, 133, 135
Urine, 26

Varicose veins, 68, 79, 113, 132
Vegan, 41–43, 47, 154
Vegetarian, 16, 40–43, 45–46, 48–49, 51–54
Vilcabamba, 166

Vitamin, 11–12, 17, 18, 24–25, 38, 40, 47, 49, 80–87, 90, 92, 102–9, 175
Vitamins (specific):
A, 19, 25, 89, 99, 103, 104, 105, 109, 143, 155
B group (see also Biotin, Choline, Inositol, Niacin, Pantothenic acid, Pyridoxine, Riboflavin, Thiamine), 25, 26–27, 31, 44, 88, 95–97, 98, 99, 100, 101, 105–7, 116, 131, 133, 134, 143, 152, 154, 167
B₁ (see Thiamine)
B₂ (see Riboflavin)
B₆ (see Pyridoxine)
B₁₂, 43, 105, 119
C, 25, 33, 49, 54, 82, 87, 88, 95, 98, 99, 100, 103, 109, 111–12, 143, 154, 160, 167, 173
D, 20, 24, 25, 87, 88, 89, 99, 103, 104, 105, 109, 116–17, 143, 154, 159, 164
E, 25, 28, 32, 82, 83, 87, 88, 89, 90, 92, 94, 95, 99, 100, 103, 107, 112–28, 123, 124, 129, 132, 135, 137, 143, 155, 158, 159, 164, 165, 178
K, 25, 87, 88, 99, 134
P, 112, 143, 154

Water Cure, 38

Wheat germ, 44, 92, 94, 107, 110, 132, 150, 155

Whole food, 16, 40, 55–56, 62–63, 149, 161, 163, 168, 172

Yeast, 44, 107, 155, 165

Yoghurt, 44, 152–53, 155, 158

Yudkin, John, 23, 36, 65, 70–73, 75, 161, 166